IN PURSUIT OF PREGNANCY

IN PURSUIT OF PREGNANCY

HOW COUPLES DISCOVER, COPE WITH, AND RESOLVE THEIR FERTILITY PROBLEMS

JOAN LIEBMANN-SMITH

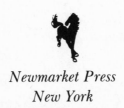

Newmarket Press
New York

First Edition
87 88 89 90 91   10 9 8 7 6 5 4 3 2 1 hc

Library of Congress Cataloging-in-Publication Data

Liebmann-Smith, Joan.
In pursuit of pregnancy.

Bibliography: p.
Includes index.
1. Infertility—Popular works.   I. Title.
RC889.L54   1987   616.6'92   86-28656
ISBN 0-937858-88-9

QUANTITY PURCHASES

Companies, professional groups, clubs and other organizations may qualify
for special terms when ordering quantities of this title. For information,
contact the Special Sales Department, Newmarket Press, 18 East 48th
Street, New York, New York 10017. Phone (212) 832-3575.

Book design by Ruth Kolbert

Manufactured in the United States of America

To the memory of my parents,
John and Dorothy Liebmann

CONTENTS

FOREWORD

As individuals, we are the sum total of all our attributes—our physical and emotional characteristics, our occupations, our accomplishments. For some, this includes the ability to have children; for others, it does not. Like the color of our hair, being infertile is only a single aspect of our lives, not the one that defines who or what we are. But it has a way of making us lose sight of the larger picture.

Infertility is something that happens to whole human beings and addressing it requires more than just treating the body. Research has carried reproductive medicine to the point where we can help an astonishing number of infertile couples to have children. Yet, providing support and direction for couples is just as critical as using the latest medical treatment.

This book is about infertility. It is about coping and living with a problem over which we have very little control. It tells us what real people who have gone through this feel like. It offers tactics, secrets, and methods of dealing with problems that in many ways are absolutely unique to fertility. It lets them know that they are not alone in their suffering. It reminds them that there is a larger picture.

As a certified subspecialist in reproductive endocrinology in private practice, as well as the medical director of an *in vitro* fertilization program, I have spent most of my professional life treating infertile couples. From my daily contact with these men and women, it is clear to me that the kind of information offered in these chapters is essential to the ultimate successful resolution of infertility, whether they end up conceiving a child or not.

Though we all need support, it is difficult to find a caring friend, relative, doctor, or support group at every instant that help is needed. This book offers that help. *In Pursuit of Pregnancy* is like having a nonjudgmental, infinitely caring friend between two covers, available whenever the need arises.

For some people, this book will be the beginning of open communication about their infertility. It will be the stimulus needed to go out and join a support group like RESOLVE. For others, *In Pursuit of Pregnancy* offers the hope of an answer to their problems; it will provide the private support needed to carry a couple through the trying process of treatment. For still others, it will offer the intermittent shoring up needed between counseling sessions and medical therapy.

Like all patients, infertility patients should not be passive participants in their medical treatment. There are times when the choices involved will appear overwhelming, and it seems we must let someone else make important decisions for us. Yet, medical treatment should be a cooperative venture between patient and physician. This book shows couples how such a cooperative effort can take place, so that treatment becomes something that is done *for* and *with* them, rather than *to* them.

Whether we read this book because we ourselves have a fertility problem, or because we care about somebody who does, it offers us all a unique opportunity to look into the lives and minds of infertile men and women. In their own words, they describe the impact of infertility on their physical, social, and sexual lives. We get to know them—as individuals, and as families seeking fulfillment. We understand their frustrations, their fears, and their triumphs. They are our friends, our neighbors, our relatives, and, at times, ourselves.

Because it contributes so much to our understanding of the emotional side of infertility, *In Pursuit of Pregnancy* stands as a unique and necessary companion to the other volumes providing more scientific information for infertile couples. It is an excellent book that provides the support and reassurance needed for the completion of appropriate medical therapy and the resolution of a couple's fertility problem.

JOHN J. STANGEL, M.D.
Program Medical Director,
IVF Australia (USA),
Ltd. at United Hospital
Port Chester, NY
Private practice in
Rye, NY

PREFACE

Back in the late 1970s when my husband and I had a fertility problem, infertility wasn't yet out of the closet; there were few books and even fewer opportunities to discuss with other couples what we were going through. One of the few books I found on the subject was Barbara Eck Menning's *Infertility: A Guide for the Childless Couple* (Prentice-Hall, 1977). I read and reread that book. It was not so much the medical information that interested me; rather, it was the quotations from *real people* with fertility problems that I couldn't seem to get enough of. Here were other people expressing what I was feeling. For the first time I realized that the intense emotions I was experiencing were the same emotions other infertile women experienced. I no longer felt alone in my misery—nor did I feel my reactions were crazy or bizarre. Those anonymous voices were my first support group.

At the same time I was pursuing pregnancy, I was also pursuing a doctoral degree in sociology at the Graduate Center of the City University of New York. When it came time to choose a dissertation topic, I realized I couldn't go through with my original plan—to study breast-feeding women on a postpartum unit. I was in no shape to deal with nursing mothers.

What interested me instead was infertility. I constantly read about it, talked about it, and obsessed about it. It seemed like a natural for a dissertation topic, since I was both personally and professionally interested in the subject. And I thought that by approaching the subject from a sociological perspective, I could gain some objectivity and make my obsession work *for* me rather than against me. I settled on the topic "Delayed Childbearing and Infertility." My obsessive reading and talking to others with fertility problems became "data collection" and laid the groundwork for my dissertation research and, later, this book.

When I decided to write a book that I hoped would help couples cope with the many crises of infertility, I thought back to what I wanted to read and needed to hear. I realized that I wanted to know more about the people behind the quotations. I wanted more details—who they were, how they coped, how they resolved their infertility. So I decided that my book would include not only quotations from real people, but also the personal journeys of several couples from the discovery of their fertility problems to their resolution.

After much thought and discussion with friends who were or had been infertile, I decided to choose three couples who had had varying types of fertility problems and had sought different solutions. Of course, I couldn't include each medical or emotional problem, nor could I interview couples of every socioeconomic class. But I thought I could find couples whose experiences were representative of what most infertile couples went through, and who could verbally express their thoughts and feelings about it.

I then called people I knew who were personally or professionally involved with infertile couples and asked if they might know any couples who had fairly typical fertility problems and who had been able to resolve those problems to their satisfaction. They would also have to be willing to be interviewed at length for the book.

I obtained the names of several couples who agreed to talk to me. I interviewed them on the phone and explained that I would like to have several in-depth interviews with both husband and wife simultaneously, as a couple. I believed this was very important; infertility is very much a couples' problem, and I hoped the dialogue between the spouses would be helpful to other couples. I assured them that their names and other identifying facts would be changed to protect their privacy.

Luckily, after not too many calls I came up with three ideal couples—Roy and Mai Li, Anthony and Sue, and Eric and Lisa (not their real names). They all had different problems and had found different solutions—and were willing to be interviewed as couples. All three agreed not for the possible publicity, since they all would have pseudonyms, but in order to share their experiences, both positive and negative, in the hope that they could help other infertile couples.

The interviews were emotionally intense for us all. In recounting their experiences, the couples often had to relive many things they would sooner have forgotten. My own often forgotten experiences with infertility vividly came back to me. There were lots of tears— and laughter. I am deeply grateful to each of these couples for allowing me to probe into some of the most personal aspects of their lives, and for, at times, disturbing their peace.

I also want to thank each of the more than fifty other men and women who over the past several years allowed me to interview them. Their quotations are scattered throughout the book to illustrate various points. Their names and other facts have also been changed to protect their identities. Although their stories are as interesting and important as those of the three main couples, it would have been impossible to include them all in detail.

One other couple's contribution was especially valuable to the writing of this book. I want to thank Larry and Sarah Madison for their word processor—without which I would still be retyping.

Many other people helped me with this book. My agent, Felicia Eth, formerly of Writers House, provided me with invaluable help in writing the proposal. She also persevered in finding the right publisher, Newmarket Press. Ann Edelstein, who took over after Felicia went to California, has also been very helpful.

I wish to thank Esther Margolis, publisher of Newmarket, who believed in this book and had the confidence that I could write it. Remmel Nunn and Theresa Burns at Newmarket not only did a fine job editing, but constantly encouraged me and provided me with the positive reinforcement I needed to complete the book.

I would also like to thank Beverly Freeman of RESOLVE and John Stangel, M.D., for their time, input, and helpful suggestions. Loren Greene, M.D., Sharon Lewin, M.D., Margaret Weiss, M.S.W., and Joyce Zeitz of the American Fertility Society have all made valuable contributions to this book.

Diane Clapp, B.S.N., R.N., Kate Gorman, D.S.W., Miriam Mazor, M.D., Roselle Shubin, M.S.W., Machalle Seibel, M.D., Sherman Silber, M.D., and Edward Wallach, M.D., were also kind enough to share their professional expertise.

I also wish to thank Samuel Bloom, Ph.D., Patricia Kendall, Ph.D., and Barbara Kats Rothman, Ph.D., for encouraging me in my career as both a sociologist and a writer.

Cathy Travis and Caroline Helmuth did a wonderful job transcribing sometimes inaudible tapes.

Special thanks to Pat Dewar for making herself available many times when she probably had better things to do. She provided me with precious hours while providing loving care for the most precious thing in my life—my daughter, Rebecca. And I want to thank Rebecca for her patience and understanding while Mommy was writing a book that would help people who were trying very hard to become mommies and daddies.

Most of all, I want to thank my husband, Richard, the best editor I know, for his loving support, understanding, and editorial comments. Without his help I could never have written this book.

And finally, very special thanks to Dr. Sami David, who helped us in our own pursuit of pregnancy.

The following couples are real people, although their names and certain other identifying facts have been changed for reasons of confidentiality. Their stories will be told throughout this book.

THE COOPERS

Roy and Mai Li Cooper met at a San Francisco party and fell in love. They weren't married, however, for another four years. Two years into their marriage, they decided to try to have a baby. After many frustrating months, they discovered that Mai Li had a medical disorder that was preventing her from conceiving.

Roy is 41-year-old cinematographer. Mai Li, who is Chinese-American, is thirty-one and a sportswear buyer.

THE SPANELLIS

Anthony and Sue Spanelli waited until they were both in their mid-thirties before they got married, but then decided to get pregnant immediately so they could have two children by the time Sue was thirty-eight. But things did not work out for them as planned—they both turned out to have fertility problems.

Anthony, thirty-nine, is from an immigrant Italian family. He is a computer programmer. Sue, also thirty-nine, is a psychologist and originally from the Midwest.

THE FELDMANS

Lisa and Eric Feldman had both been quite wild when they first met back in the sixties. When they remet in the eighties, they decided to settle down, get married, and raise a family. In fact, they were both so intent on starting their family they tried to conceive before the wedding. But like the Coopers and Spanellis, they discovered they were infertile.

Lisa, thirty, is a secretary. Eric is a thirty-six-year-old orthopedic surgeon.

CHAPTER 1

*I really thought I was going to get pregnant on the first try.
When the fifth month came I was a basket case because it
wasn't happening. Then one month my period was two-and-a-
half weeks late, which it never is. And I thought for sure,
so I had a pregnancy test. I wasn't pregnant. I felt like I had
had a miscarriage. I was so overcome, I just sobbed
and sobbed.*

TRYING
TO GET PREGNANT
–AND NOT SUCCEEDING

THE COOPERS

Roy and Mai Li met in San Francisco at a party given by a mutual friend. Mai Li was with her date, a married man she had been seeing for two years. She was twenty-three and interested in meeting other men because she realized her relationship with the married man was going nowhere. Roy had just broken up with his girl friend of several years. He came over to Mai Li and introduced himself.

MAI LI: I took one look at Roy and it was love at first sight! He was really good-looking and had a wonderful sense of humor. I immediately asked him his age and whether he was married. He was thirty-three and single. I couldn't believe my good fortune—I had finally met Mr. Right. But my date came over, and Roy walked away.

1

ROY: I really liked Mai Li, but I had just gotten out of one stormy relationship and didn't want to move in on anyone else's territory, so I didn't ask for her telephone number.

MAI LI: I couldn't stop thinking about him. I knew he was a filmmaker, so I looked him up in the Yellow Pages. He had told me at the party that he was moving into a new apartment, so I called him up under the pretense that I was looking for an apartment and was interested in his old apartment. He said I couldn't have his apartment because it was a sublet, and then he asked me out to dinner.

ROY: We dated for two years and lived together for another two years. Mai Li was always bugging me to get married, but I wasn't ready to settle down. One Saturday I went to spend the day in the country with a friend and his two sons. It was wonderful. I came home and said to Mai Li, "Let's get married and have kids."

Roy and Mai Li got married when she was twenty-six and he was thirty-six. By then, Roy was a successful filmmaker and Mai Li was a sportswear buyer for a large department store. Two years after they got married, they decided to have a baby.

ROY: When we got married we wrote our own marriage vows, and one of the things I said was that I was looking forward to raising a family with Mai Li. It never occurred to either one of us that Mai Li would not get pregnant within a reasonable period of time. We thought it might even happen the first month we tried. After all, we had been using birth control for years.

MAI LI: I didn't think there would be a problem at all. When it didn't happen the first month I didn't think it was a big deal—that it certainly would happen in a month or two. But when it went into three and four months I started to become alarmed. Even though it was early to get alarmed, I had kind of a—I don't know whether I was fatalistic or it was a premonition—but I had a sense that something was wrong.

ROY: I certainly didn't have the same alarmed attitude that Mai Li had about the length of time it was taking us to get pregnant. But when she decided to pursue what she thought was a problem, I felt ambivalent. It's one of the areas where Mai Li so closely resembles my mother, although my mother is Jewish and my wife Chinese-American. So I always take these things with a grain of salt—I'm conditioned to live with that. When my father died of a heart attack, my mother got a phone call telling her the bad news. She had expected that call for thirty-five years. When it finally came, she said, "I knew it!" And Mai Li is a lot like my mother. And yet I couldn't help having a double or triple reaction to her anxiety: one, you're crazy, it's only three months; two, oh, my God, what if she's right; and three, OK, let's be rational and sensible about this and keep it in check.

MAI LI: I had convinced myself that it was Roy's problem. The minute I found out that there might be a problem, I started reading about infertility, and I had read some statistics about the age of the man being a factor, so I was concerned about Roy since he was forty.

ROY: Mai Li read that excessive heat around the scrotum could inhibit sperm development, so she went out and bought me boxer shorts and I wore them faithfully. I also stopped taking hot baths and showers. Once I had to go on location in Denver and one of the shots we had to do was in a hot tub and I couldn't even go in!

MAI LI: Roy's a very cooperative guy. And I was extremely impatient and aggressive about this, so rather than wait six more months for a semen analysis, I convinced Roy to do it after two more months.

ROY: The morning I had to go there, Mai Li couldn't come with me. I was very anxious. I had my jar and my paper bag and was "white knuckling" the paper bag because I had fantasies of dropping it and spilling my sperm all over the place. The office turned out to be in the sub-subterranean basement of a medical center. The whole thing reeked of a Boris Karloff movie—I go in there with my jar expecting this nurse, who had a German accent on the phone, to be an ancient German lady. I walked in and there was this young, beautiful blonde. Now I was anxious *and* embarrassed. But the doctor was terrific—he had a double-sided microscope so the patients could also see their sperm. He said, "There are lots of them buggers in there." I was fine—and relieved.

MAI LI: My doctor next suggested that I start keeping a temperature chart to see if I ovulated. The next step would be to have a hysterosalpingogram—they would shoot dye into my [fallopian] tubes and x-ray them to see if they were blocked.

From the moment I went to my doctor and said, "Hey, there might be a problem," that was the first step in accepting the reality that I had a problem. So when reality hit, I was somewhat prepared. I was not shot in the back—I saw it coming.

Roy and Mai Li are not alone. In fact, an estimated one couple in six in the United States is infertile—that is, they are unable to conceive or carry a pregnancy to term after one year of trying. Infertility should not be confused with sterility, which is the absolute inability to reproduce. Most infertile couples are not, in fact, sterile. Statistics now suggest that infertility is on the rise. This is thought to be due to several factors: the increase in the use of intrauterine devices (IUDs), the number of abortions, *in vitro* exposure to diethylstilbestrol (DES), the high incidence of venereal diseases, and the larger number of women who have delayed childbearing until their mid- to late thirties. In addition, environmental factors, such as toxic chemicals and radiation exposure, are believed to have contributed to an increase in the incidence of infertility.

A FALSE SENSE OF SECURITY

Most couples, like Roy and Mai Li, assume they are fertile and that when they want to, they'll be able to conceive almost instantly. Indeed, many people spend much of their single years (or early married years) concerned with *avoiding* pregnancy. For them, fertility is something they never question.

I was certain it would happen the first month. After all, my wife had gotten pregnant with an IUD and had to have an abortion. We thought we were super-fertile!

Some couples, like the above, who had no trouble conceiving one child, may find that they have "secondary infertility" and can't conceive another. And some people who have had a child with their ex-spouses find that they are infertile with their new spouse.

Many women have a false sense of security about childbearing because they have always been basically healthy.

When I put that diaphragm away, I was ready to get pregnant that very month. Infertility was one health problem that I never dreamed of having. I always thought that I was very fertile—I'm physically very voluptuous, and I got my period when I was eleven. I never skipped a period. Everything about my biological system seemed to work according to the textbook. I had no previous history of any kind of "female complaints," no infections, no previous abortion, no miscarriages. I went to the gynecologist for a routine exam every year. In fact, before I started trying, I asked my doctor if he could check me out to see if I might have any problems conceiving. He gave me an internal and said, "Everything's normal. Go out and get pregnant"—that was three years ago!

Unfortunately, the doctor inadvertently misled this woman. A doctor cannot possibly determine whether a couple is fertile just by doing an internal exam. In fact, the only definitive proof of fertility is a pregnancy. So, even if a couple has had a previous pregnancy, they have no way of knowing whether they can become pregnant again until they actually do become pregnant.

FACING THE POSSIBILITY OF A PROBLEM

How couples come to terms with the possibility of a fertility problem varies tremendously. Very often the wife is the first to express concern—after all, she is the one who will or will not become pregnant. She is also the one who monitors her body and looks for signs of pregnancy or impending menstruation, and she may misinterpret the signs for either.

The first month we tried, I just knew I was pregnant. I felt different. I read about women saying "I just knew this was the night I conceived," and I have often had feelings like that. I now know that I can't trust a single thing except not getting a period for at least three weeks.

Facing the possibility of a fertility problem is extremely difficult at best, and some try to put off finding out the truth for as long as possible.

The doctor I was going to when I got rid of my IUD said, "Give yourself at least a year on your own. And after a year if you still haven't conceived, we'll start the tests." Well, I pushed a year into a year and a half and into a year and three-quarters because I couldn't face both the thought of the testing, which I knew was very painful, and the idea of finding out that I was infertile.

A woman not only has to come to terms with the possibility of infertility, but she often has to convince her husband that there might be a problem. Many husbands have a more difficult time accepting this than do their wives.

My wife was the first one to think there was a problem. I kept saying that it usually takes six months to a year, and I kept delaying doing anything, saying, "It's OK, it doesn't matter." Later she was very angry about that. I was dealing with it by denial while my wife was ready to see it as a problem much sooner than I was. Emotionally it was a problem for me, although I wouldn't admit it.

A sense of humor helps some couples come to terms with their situation.

There is a sample temperature chart that comes with the basal thermometer, and this fictional woman has such a nice, clean ovulation. It goes along nicely and then dips and shoots up again, and you can see on day fourteen that she ovulated. But my charts always had this zigzag line—we'd look at the chart together and compare my chart with hers and laugh. We laughed until we got to the point where it really wasn't funny any more.

The realization that a problem may exist is the first in a long succession of crises you are likely to face. It will help if you try to understand each other's fears, doubts, insecurities, guilt, and anger that typically accompany infertility. And perhaps most importantly, you should remember that infertility is a couple's problem, and the best way for you to deal with it is by confronting it together.

THE SPANELLIS

Anthony and Sue met in a creative writing class. Sue had recently arrived in New York from the Midwest, where she had lived her whole life, to complete her education as a psychologist. Anthony, the son of Italian immigrants, had been born and raised in the city. He was a computer programmer. The first time they spoke to each other was in the subway.

> ANTHONY: I was running to catch the subway and noticed this attractive woman from my writing class getting in the subway car, so I rushed down real fast to catch her and made it into the car just as the doors were closing. I sat in the seat directly in front of her and tried to look nice and suave. I ignored her for several stops and then started talking to her, but I didn't ask her out until after our next class. Then I asked her out for a cup of coffee before my yoga class. I was very into classes in those days!
>
> SUE: We dated a long time before we really got serious, and waited five years before we decided to get married. We were from very different backgrounds, and we wanted to be certain that we had a good relationship and would have a good marriage. We really took the time to work out any problems, so that when issues came up, we'd have the tools to deal with them.

They finally decided to get married when they were both thirty-five, because at that point they were ready to start their family.

ANTHONY: I saw no reason why we couldn't get pregnant fairly quickly. I thought, Well, we're both healthy, so there was no reason why we shouldn't.

SUE: We just thought people got pregnant right away. Also I had things all planned out in my mind for the next several years, and having children was part of that plan. I wanted to change jobs at a certain time, finish my doctorate, and have two children by the time I was thirty-eight years old.

But after several months, I still wasn't pregnant and began to get very concerned. I was already thirty-six. I went to my gynecologist for a routine checkup, but I really wanted to find out whether or not I should be concerned. My doctor recommended that Anthony have a semen analysis.

ANTHONY: I was not anticipating any problems at all. I thought the semen analysis was just a formality to make sure nothing is wrong—something routine to cover all bases, nothing to really worry about.

SUE: My doctor called me up at home on a Sunday and said, "I've got the results of the semen analysis, and I don't like how it looks." I was surprised and felt sort of panicky—Oh, God! We have a problem!

ANTHONY: Sue got off the phone and told me that something was wrong with my sperm. I froze—I was very upset. Part of it was the fear of the unknown. I thought, What could possibly be wrong with me? Did I have a venereal disease I didn't know about? Had I been exposed to radiation? Even my Roman Catholic morality began creeping in, and I thought maybe I did something really wrong—I probably masturbated too much as a teenager and this was God's punishment.

WHAT IS NECESSARY FOR CONCEPTION TO TAKE PLACE?

In order to understand why pregnancy doesn't happen, it helps to understand how pregnancy does occur. Here is a very simplified description of how conception takes place.

- The woman must ovulate a healthy, ripe, fertilizable egg at midcycle.

- Her fallopian tubes must be open in order to receive the egg.
- The couple must have intercourse within twenty-four to forty-eight hours of ovulation.
- The man must ejaculate healthy sperm in adequate numbers deep into the woman's vagina.
- The sperm must travel through the cervix into the uterus and finally into the fallopian tubes.
- The egg must be fertilized by the sperm in a fallopian tube and then travel down to the uterus.
- The egg must implant itself in a normally shaped, hormonally primed uterus and grow into a healthy embryo.

You can see there is lots of room for something to go wrong—and it often does. For example, women do not ovulate every single month; most normal women miss at least one ovulation each year. In fact, a healthy young couple trying to conceive have only a 20 percent chance each month of being successful. In other words, they really only have a good chance of getting pregnant in one out of five months of trying. If you are a woman in your late twenties to early thirties, your chances each month drop to around 10 to 15 percent. And if you're in your late thirties, the chances are under 10 percent each month. This explains why it takes the average couple six months to a year to conceive.

Both men and women are most fertile when they are in their mid-twenties. After thirty, fertility for women starts to decline slowly until about age thirty-five, when it begins to decline rather rapidly. Male fertility steadily but slowly declines after age forty. Statistically, the younger you are, the better are your chances of conceiving. This doesn't mean that if you are in your thirties you won't ever get pregnant; it just may take longer, or you may have a fertility problem that requires medical attention.

Never in my wildest dreams did I think we'd have trouble, even though I was thirty-eight and my husband forty. A woman once asked me when I was going to have children. And I said, "I don't know; there's time." And she said very casually, "Well, you know, it might not be so easy. You might have problems." And I just flicked it out of my mind. I thought that the minute I put my mind to it, it would happen. I'm now forty-three; I had one miscarriage and I'm still trying.

DECIDING TO CONSULT A DOCTOR

Most couples finally consult a doctor after much thought and discussion, and with a sense of relief. Now some of the burden can be shared—it is up to the doctor to find out what's wrong and to help the couple get pregnant.

Once the decision is made to consult a doctor, the couple is usually ready for action. They expect tests, a diagnosis, and a prognosis. If for any reason the doctor does not perceive their difficulty in getting pregnant as a problem, the couple is likely to feel frustrated and annoyed, if not confused.

> The doctor was very relaxed, and his whole attitude was very relaxed. He never gave me the feeling that it was a terribly urgent thing that I must immediately check out. He kept saying, "We'll wait a few more months and see"—he said, "Maybe you should take a vacation."

This woman was thirty-seven. Unfortunately, she waited another year before going back to her doctor for tests, wasting precious time. It is true that many doctors wait a year before starting a fertility workup on most couples, but most fertility specialists agree that if you are a woman in your thirties, you should probably see a fertility specialist after trying for only six months. Whatever your age, before you consult a doctor it's a good idea to start keeping a temperature chart to help determine whether or not you ovulate. (See BBT below.)

> About a year and a half after we started trying to get pregnant my husband said, "We're trying to get pregnant much in the same way we do lots of things—without looking into it very well and just sort of trusting that it was going to happen without even knowing what we were doing. And it clearly isn't happening, so why don't we take some tests or do something about it?" Then he said, "Why don't you go buy a

thermometer?" And I said, "A thermometer? What do I need a thermometer for?" I had no idea! And he said, "Don't you know anything about your own ovulation?" I said, "Not a thing." I knew nothing, nothing.

If you have any suspicion or fear that you or your spouse may have a fertility problem—and I assume you do if you are reading this book—if you haven't yet consulted a physician, you should certainly do so; you have nothing to lose. And, if possible, it would be preferable to see a fertility specialist (see chapter 2 for information on how to find one). The specialist may be able to provide some reassurance while obtaining basic information by starting with several simple, noninvasive tests.

Preliminary Fertility Tests

Semen analysis. This is the easiest test for the husband. He masturbates to produce a semen sample and brings it to a lab or a urologist for analysis. The sperm are counted to make sure there are enough for fertilization to occur. The activity level of the sperm (motility) is measured to see what percentage are moving and what percentage are inactive. The shape of the sperm (morphology) is also evaluated to see what percentage are normal and what percentage are abnormally shaped. The volume of the semen is also measured, and it is checked for bacteria that may interfere with fertility.

Basal body temperature (BBT). This is the easiest test for the wife. It involves keeping a daily record of her temperature upon awakening in the morning. Charting her temperature fluctuations keeps track of the length of her menstrual cycle and helps determine whether she ovulates.

Blood hormone levels. Both men and women should have their blood tested to determine if they have normal levels of hormones. Men are usually tested for testosterone, follicle-stimulating hormone (FSH), and lutenizing hormone (LH), all three of which are necessary for sperm production. Women are also commonly tested for FSH, LH, and testosterone as well as estrogen, progesterone, and prolactin. These hormones all play an important role in pregnancy. Both men and women should also have their thyroid levels tested, because an under- or overactive thyroid can interfere with fertility.

Postcoital test. For this test, the couple has intercourse as close to ovulation as possible. At this time the woman's cervical mucus is more easily penetrated by the sperm. Several hours after intercourse, the woman goes to the doctor's office and has her cervical mucus examined under a microscope to determine how well the sperm have survived. This very important test can reveal problems with the cervical mucus, the sperm, and the interaction of both.

Tests for infections. Both partners should be tested for T-*Mycoplasma* and *Chlamydia*, both of which are fairly common bacteria that cause infections which can interfere with fertility.

The above tests should be done before you have any of the following routine, informative, but more invasive procedures:

Endometrial biopsy. A few days after ovulation, a small piece of the lining of the uterus (endometrium) is cut out and examined under a microscope. The progesterone level is then measured. This is a very accurate way of determining whether a woman has ovulated, as well as whether she has adequate amounts of progesterone to sustain a pregnancy. This test can be somewhat painful, but the pain usually lasts only a few minutes at the most. You may find it helpful to take anticramp medication such as Motrin ahead of time to help alleviate the pain.

There is some controversy over when this procedure should be done. There is evidence that if it is done after ovulation, and the woman has conceived, it can cause a miscarriage. Also, some specialists believe that they can get more information from the biopsy if it is done at the very end of the menstrual cycle.

Hysterosalpingogram. This procedure is usually done in a radiologist's office. Radiopaque dye is injected through the cervix into the fallopian tubes and uterus. This helps determine whether the tubes are blocked and whether the uterus is shaped normally. The woman may feel mild to severe cramping from this procedure. Taking an anticramp medication such as Motrin before the procedure can help lessen the pain.

Laparoscopy. Laparoscopy is a surgical technique in which the doctor inserts a telescopelike instrument called a laparoscope through the navel to inspect the ovaries, fallopian tubes, and uterus visually. This procedure provides very accurate information about these organs and is the best way to determine whether there are any adhesions—bands of scar tissue that extend from one organ surface to another—that may be causing the infertility. Because laparoscopy is a surgical procedure that involves the use of general anesthesia, there are certain risks involved that you should discuss with your physician.

There are many other tests and procedures your doctor might recommend. Included in the appendix is a list of excellent books written by fertility specialists for infertile couples. In them you will find detailed descriptions of all the different procedures, as well as information about the causes of and treatments for most fertility problems.

THE FELDMANS

Lisa and Eric first met back in the sixties when Lisa was twenty and Eric twenty-six. Ten years later, Lisa broke her foot in a skiing accident; her internist referred her to an orthopedic surgeon—Eric. According to Lisa, "I told him I couldn't possibly use him as a doctor after we had done drugs together in the sixties." Although he couldn't convince her to become his patient, he did convince her to go out with him. Said Eric, "We knew we loved each other from the first day we went out. And we knew something was going to come of it." They were married six months later because they both wanted children right away. In fact, they decided to try to get pregnant before the wedding.

LISA: I knew I would get pregnant right away—I absolutely knew it. And two months later, I really thought I was pregnant.

ERIC: Lisa was always very regular—on the dot. She could tell days before her period because she would start cleaning. This month the apartment was filthy, and she was ten days late.

LISA: My father was very, very sick at that point and we had to take him to the emergency room. When we got there, I went to the bathroom. I had gotten my period. I was devastated.

ERIC: We knew something was wrong then. I spoke to a colleague who suggested I get tested first and recommended a urologist who specialized in male infertility. I made the call, but I really didn't want to believe that it could be my problem. I had always had a feeling that I was fertile, because there was a woman in my past who had told me I was responsible for her pregnancy. So I thought, It can't be me. It was the one thing I thought I was good at—that was my macho self.

LISA: We always had a lot of family jokes about Eric's private parts being very large—from the time he was a baby, his family used to make fun of that. And he is very masculine and very hairy, so I was sure it wasn't him.

ERIC: There was something about Lisa that was very female, very fertile; I felt it couldn't be her. The minute I made that first call to the doctor—that was the admission that I was going to find out that it was me.

LISA: I was certain it was me. First of all, it's always the woman. Secondly, there is a big history in my family of fertility problems. Plus, when I was a teenager, I had gotten pregnant a few times and the doctor who did the abortions had said, "Young lady, if you keep this up, you're not going to be able to have children when you want them." That's why I was convinced it was me.

ERIC: I always had horrible experiences with doctors; every time I go they find something wrong. That's probably why I went into medicine—to gain some control over my own health.

I walked into the doctor's office for an eight-thirty-A.M. appointment and there were, it seemed like, four hundred people in the waiting room—it was like the whole world had a fertility problem! Dr. B. told me that everything was off—count, morphology, and motility. But since there were some viable sperm, he said I was considered subfertile, not sterile. He thought I might have a varicocele—an enlarged vein in the testicle. So I had this wild exam where he was down by my testicles and I had to blow very hard, but he didn't find a varicocele. Then he showed me his "scrotum necklace"—rings of all different sizes to measure testicles! He said that perhaps the problem was my profession—that I might have been exposed to too much radiation.

LISA: When Eric came home that night, we sat down on the couch and he said, "It's me." We both cried. I was really shocked—I had been so convinced it was my problem.

ERIC: We both hugged each other. We cried for a minute and said, "Now what do we do?" I really needed Lisa a lot at that point. I really needed to be cared for. She was very strong about it—her attitude was, this should be our worst problem. Let's go on from here.

WHOSE PROBLEM IS IT ANYWAY?

Until recently infertility was almost always thought to be the fault of the woman. In certain cultures, a barren marriage is even considered adequate grounds for a man to divorce his wife. In fact, in at least two-thirds of the cases of infertility, the man either exclusively has the problem, or both husband and wife have a combined problem. Only one-third of the time is the problem solely the wife's. And just because one spouse is found to have a problem doesn't mean the other should be medically ignored. The spouse without the diagnosed problem may in fact turn out to have a problem that was overlooked, or may subsequently develop a fertility problem.

The discovery of an actual fertility problem is a major crisis for most couples. Whether or not they have an initial diagnosis, they are usually shocked that they are about to seek medical intervention for something they thought would come naturally. They are finally forced to face the reality of their situation— that they are infertile. Every step of the way, from the realization of a problem to the resolution of the infertility, the couple is continuously confronted with new crises. In the next chapter we will see how the Coopers, the Spanellis, and the Feldmans dealt with the medical crisis of infertility and handled the doctor-patient relationship.

CHAPTER 2

Oh, my first doctor I adored. He was a very kind, sensitive, wonderful, dedicated person. But infertility was not his field of expertise, and after a while I thought he was just futzing around.

DEALING WITH DOCTORS

THE SPANELLIS

After the initial shock of finding out that Anthony had a fertility problem, the couple made an appointment to see his urologist. He told them that Anthony's sperm count was good, but he had poor morphology and motility. He then examined Anthony. "It's unmistakable," he said. "You have bilateral varicoceles." He explained that this meant that Anthony had enlarged (varicose) veins on both his testicles. About 10 percent of all men have varicoceles, usually on the left side, and most varicoceles do not cause fertility problems. However, they are one of the most common causes of male infertility. It is believed that they interfere with sperm production because they heat up the scrotum and kill some sperm and cause others to be misshapen.

The urologist ran more tests on Anthony and recommended a varicocelectomy, a surgical procedure that would remove the varicoceles. He explained that it could take up to a year to show some improvement—and he warned that in about 30 percent of cases, there is no improvement. Anthony decided to go ahead with the operation. While they were waiting to see if the operation had improved Anthony's sperm, the urologist suggested that they do husband inseminations (AIH)—that is, artificial insemination with Anthony's sperm. Three months after his surgery, Anthony was retested. The operation had been a success. However, Anthony's doctor still thought they should continue the inseminations.

ANTHONY: Dr. T., Sue's gynecologist, thought the inseminations were a waste of time but agreed to do it because my doctor had recommended them.

SUE: I had a lot of confidence in Dr. T. I thought she would be a good doctor because a friend of mine who recommended her thought she was wonderful and a lot of her friends went to her and liked her, although none had fertility problems. I really trusted her. She said to me, "If you stick with me, you'll get pregnant." But month after month I still wasn't getting pregnant. I thought there had to be something wrong with me, since Anthony's sperm were now fine.

Dr. T. turned out to be a very poor doctor. I was not tested for over a year—no blood tests, no postcoitals, nothing, nothing. She only had me keep temperature charts because I was having artificial inseminations and taking a fertility drug, Clomid. I kept going to her because she had convinced me that she knew exactly what she was doing and how to treat infertility. She finally decided to do a laparoscopy. I was nervous about her doing it, but I felt something had to be done. I hadn't read a thing, so I knew nothing about the whole range of tests that should be done before a laparoscopy. She found only a few small fibroids, benign growths in my uterus, but didn't think they were preventing me from getting pregnant.

When I did finally question something she did, she was indignant. I have cycles where it's very unpredictable when I ovulate, even on Clomid. But she thought there should not be individual variations—she thought my cycles should be twenty-eight-day cycles. When I expressed concern about her timing of the inseminations she said, "The twenty-eight-day cycle is an international standard—what do you mean by saying your cycles are not twenty-eight days?" She had been getting my temperature charts by that time for at least a year and a half and I don't think she ever looked at them! My cycles were anywhere from twenty-four to thirty-five days, and it was right there on my temperature charts! Then she started to figure out when the next month's inseminations would be and she started counting on her fingers and must have left out a hand, she was so far off! That's when I thought of switching doctors. I thought, Oh, my God, what are we doing going to this doctor? How can somebody treat infertility when you have to fit your ovulation to their schedule? I said to Anthony, "There must be infertility specialists who deal with this kind of problem."

WHO SHOULD TREAT INFERTILITY?

Very often, the infertile couple first consults their regular gynecologist. However, the average gynecologist does not have extensive training in reproductive endocrinology and infertility. Many of these doctors recognize their limitations and may either refer the couple right away to a fertility specialist or may start the couple off by having them keep temperature charts and have simple blood tests before referring them to a specialist. However, as Sue found out, there are other nonspecialists who continue to treat the infertility patient and wind up wasting the couple's time—and money.

Of course it's not easy for a doctor to admit that he might not be an expert in an area his patient expects him to know about. The patient, too, has to take some responsibility for his or her own health care. Liking a doctor is not enough reason to continue seeing him; he should be an expert in the area where the problem exists.

According to Beverly Freeman, president of RESOLVE, Inc., a national self-help organization for infertile couples:

If someone has not achieved a pregnancy in about a year, they should see a specialist right away. Infertility is very

complicated, and only an infertility specialist is really qualified to diagnose and treat the very subtle and difficult aspects
of infertility.

But what should you do if you have already started infertility
testing and treatment with your regular gynecologist and he is
not a fertility specialist? Should you stick with him, or go to a
specialist as this woman did?

I like Dr. A., I really like him. And I don't think he treats me
in a paternalistic manner either. He treats me as an intelligent
individual, not a dumb female. I hope I'm not going to have
too much difficulty when I tell him that for my own peace of
mind I think it's better for me to go to a fertility expert, and
that I'd love to come back to him after I get pregnant.

Ms. Freeman advises:

In the event your regular gynecologist has diagnosed and
treated your problem and you are having regular intercourse
and still aren't pregnant in six to twelve cycles, a higher level
of diagnosis is called for, such as immunological studies and a
laparoscopy. For these you should move on to a fertility
specialist. However, if you are over thirty-five, you should see
a specialist straight off.

Many physicians in different specialties are trained to some
extent to deal with fertility problems. A list of the specialists
you are most likely to consult for a fertility problem follows,
but it is up to you to find out if they in fact have had additional training that qualifies them to deal with male or female
infertility.

Urologists. Physicians who specialize in the diagnosis and treatment of diseases of the reproductive organs in men and of the
urinary tract in men and women. Urologists are also trained to
perform surgery. They may or may not have advanced training
in the treatment of infertility.

Andrologists. Physicians, usually urologists, who specialize in
the male reproductive system and hormones.

Obstetrician-gynecologists (Ob-gyns). Physicians who specialize in the management of pregnancy and childbirth and in the diagnosis and treatment of diseases of women. They are qualified surgeons and may or may not have extensive training in infertility. However, if most of their practice is devoted to obstetrics (delivering babies), they usually do not have adequate time to devote to an infertility practice.

Reproductive endocrinologists. Ob-gyns who have completed a fellowship in reproductive endocrinology—two years of intensive training in infertility that focuses on the role of hormones in reproduction. Reproductive endocrinologists are also trained in microsurgery and, more recently, in *in vitro* fertilization. There are only approximately 350 certified reproductive endocrinologists in the United States.

HOW TO FIND OUT
IF A DOCTOR IS A FERTILITY SPECIALIST

Some doctors who really do not have adequate postgraduate training call themselves fertility specialists. You can and should, therefore, check your doctor's credentials to make certain you are in the hands of an expert. Edward E. Wallach, M.D., professor and chairman of the department of gynecology and obstetrics at the Johns Hopkins Medical Institutions and former president of the American Fertility Society, advises that:

—the patient with a fertility problem seek a physician who has had at least two years of postresidency training in a recognized program approved by the American Board of Obstetrics and Gynecology. The physician who is certified by the American College of Obstetrics and Gynecology as having specific competence in reproductive endocrinology has added certification of excellence. With respect to male infertility, no such certification exists. However, there are certain urologists who have expertise in the management of infertility.

—the patient inquire as to whether a physician is certified by the American Board of Obstetrics and Gynecology in reproductive endocrinology and has had a fellowship in reproductive endocrinology.

—those seeking an infertility specialist check with the American Fertility Society, RESOLVE, or the department of obstetrics and gynecology in the nearest university medical center.

In addition, you might want to ask your general practitioner (G.P.), internist, gynecologist, or friends for recommendations. Keep in mind, though, that a friend is likely to recommend a doctor who has helped *her* conceive. This does not necessarily mean that doctor is the right one for you or even qualified to treat infertility. Regardless of who recommends a fertility doctor, before you settle on one it is advisable to check the doctor's credentials with one of the above organizations.

RESOLVE's Beverly Freeman also suggests that you ask the doctor or his nurse what percentage of his practice is in infertility; she feels that at least 50 percent of the doctor's practice should be devoted to infertility. According to Ms. Freeman:

> Anyone in our view who is a specialist does a lot of infertility and little or no obstetrics. Anybody who does a lot of obstetrics probably can't pay enough attention to infertility to be considered a specialist.

If you happen to live in an area with no available fertility specialist, you should seriously consider traveling to the nearest specialist for at least one consultation. In that way, your local doctor can consult with the fertility specialist about your condition.

THE COOPERS

Mai Li followed her doctor's recommendation of keeping a temperature chart and having a hysterosalpingogram, the x-ray test of her fallopian tubes. Roy was shooting a film that day and couldn't come with her to the radiologist.

MAI LI: Two things happened that worried me—it hurt a lot, and the dye didn't pass freely through my tubes. The radiologist was very calm but said that there seemed to be a problem. I started to get very distressed. I still don't know if it was the news or the pain or a combination, but it was one big horrible experience. I went to the phone to call Roy at the film studio, and I started to cry and said, "Maybe you should come and pick me up—there's a problem." And he said, "Don't worry, we can always adopt." That was reassuring, but I didn't want to hear the word "adopt" because that was acknowledging there was a problem—another nail into the coffin, so to speak. There was no way he could leave the studio and come and get me; I was just not being rational. I just wanted to be taken care of.

I called my gynecologist the next morning to find out what was wrong. I was hoping it was all a bad dream and the hysterosalpingogram was fine, but his handling of this caused me even more alarm. He said, "Let me ask you something. Did you ever have any high fevers or infections as a child?" That approach was very distressing, because he was implying that there was a problem without saying there was a problem. It was a very roundabout way of telling me. Then I had to sit there and think of the last twenty-eight years. He said both my tubes were blocked and that the next step would be tubal repair. I said, "Are you qualified to do the surgery?" and he said, "Yes, absolutely." I said, "OK, fine," and I went to a fertility specialist instead.

ROY: It was a traumatic decision for us—I remember a lot of angst over that decision about staying with the doctor who did the diagnosis or going to another. It was the first time we ever took the initiative of being in control and saying that this person isn't good enough, and we want the best of the best. Mai Li was more forceful about that than I would have been—I would have stayed with this gynecologist and seen it through. Maybe it was timidity or a belief that he seemed qualified, and there was no reason to run off to a specialist so quickly.

MAI LI: I wanted the best. It was too sensitive and important an area to leave to my regular doctor. It was just as if I had to have surgery to reverse blindness—I would not just go to my local G.P.

I found a specialist by telling people about my problem and getting their feedback on doctors they knew or had heard about. One doctor's name kept coming up—Dr. S. We went to see him and really liked him. He agreed with the first doctor's evaluation and said he wanted to do a laparoscopy, a surgical technique that would allow him to look at my ovaries, tubes, and uterus. He said he would do laser surgery, which leads to less scarring and a quicker recovery.

I went ahead and had the laparoscopy. When I woke up from surgery he said, "I was very surprised; you were covered with endometriosis." He explained that this was a condition in which pieces of the lining of the uterus grow outside the uterus in such places as the ovaries and fallopian tubes. Endometriosis can cause pain, adhesions, and infertility, and I had all three. Dr. S. then said, "I hate this disease, but the prognosis is very, very good. I cleaned it all up."

Roy: He didn't say that to me. He told me statistically that Mai Li had a 60 percent chance of getting pregnant. I didn't consider that overly optimistic.

Mai Li: The minute I thought we might have a fertility problem, I started reading about infertility. Now that I had a diagnosed problem, I read everything I could get my hands on. I needed to feel I was on top of things—that I had some control over what was happening to me.

TAKING CHARGE OF YOUR OWN HEALTH CARE

Being in charge of your own health care is not always easy. After all, the doctor is the expert, and most of us, whether we want to or not, tend to see doctors as rather godlike authority figures. Doctors themselves are often uncomfortable with this image, yet it has persisted. They may be experts, but many doctors are overextended and cannot give all their patients their full attention—so it is up to the patients to take responsibility for their own health care.

Infertility patients are different from most patients in that they are not sick by normal definitions. They are patients only because they want, yet have been unable, to become parents. The doctor's goals and the patient's are the same—for the patient to become pregnant. How that goal is achieved depends on many factors, including just how far the patient is willing to go in order to achieve a pregnancy. The doctor may recommend a test or prescribe drugs or surgery that the patient may not want.

Tests and treatment for infertility can be unpleasant, painful, experimental, and, in some cases, even dangerous. Of course, we would like our doctors to inform us about the risks and benefits of all medical procedures, and they may do so, but it makes sense to get as much information as you can about infertility so you can ask the appropriate questions and make the correct decisions for yourself. One woman told me that when she changed doctors her new doctor recommended that she have another endometrial biopsy. When she said she would, he said, "Not so fast; you should really ask me questions. You should ask me why I want to do it again, what I expect to learn, and what the risks are."

Taking things into your own hands can also save you from unnecessary surgery, as one woman whose husband was sterile found out.

> I guess I'm one of those people who hopes the doctor is going to do his best. And I'm beginning to feel that you can't trust them—you have to almost organize your own treatment. My doctor suggested I have a laparoscopy. At first I said yes, then I went home and really thought about it. I thought, why are they fooling around with my tubes? I don't think my tubes are the problem. Just to do it because it's the last thing on the list? I felt that it wouldn't solve the problem. I just didn't want to do that, so I called and canceled it. My doctor said, "I can understand if you don't want to do that."

HOW DO YOU KNOW
IF YOUR DOCTOR IS RIGHT FOR YOU?

Most doctors are understanding and cooperative about their patients' desires to have or not to have a medical procedure. You should also be able to make suggestions to your doctor about any tests or treatments you think may be helpful. If you find that your doctor does not respond to your questions, listen to your suggestions, or respect your opinions about your fertility problem, it's time to find one who does. After all, you pay the bills—your doctor is supposed to work for, not against, you.

I'd go through my books and decide maybe this or that should be done, and I'd bring it up to him. He wasn't too happy about it. I would say, "Well, should you do some hormone testing?" And he'd say condescendingly, "Kathy, you ovulate, your hormones are not a problem." That type of thing.

This woman had another type of fairly common fertility problem—repeated miscarriages, which, contrary to what her doctor said, can be caused by a hormonal imbalance. In fact, this is the case in a small but significant percentage of miscarriages; any woman who has repeated miscarriages should have her hormones evaluated.

If you have had miscarriages, it is very important to find a doctor who knows a lot about the subject and doesn't underestimate its significance as a fertility problem.

After my second miscarriage, my doctor said he thought I had blighted ova. He said that this is something that occurs in nature, and it very possibly could occur twice in a row. When I asked if he could do some tests, he said, "There is nothing wrong with you. The only way I would give you any tests is if you had ten miscarriages!" Well, I thought it over and decided not to go back to him—it took me about thirty seconds.

RESOLVE's president, Beverly Freeman, advises that for miscarriages over and above a first very early miscarriage, you should definitely see a fertility specialist. "People don't admit that it's a fertility problem and don't understand the seriousness of it," says Ms. Freeman.

It is important to have a doctor who not only takes you seriously and can take questions, suggestions, and criticisms in stride, but who will also be available to you when you need him. If not, it is his responsibility to make provisions for an adequate backup system—either another doctor or a nurse.

After three months on the fertility drug Clomid, my doctor suggested that I take Pergonal, another, more powerful fertility drug that requires injections. He didn't really explain anything to me; he just dumped all this stuff into my hands—syringes, needles, and vials. I said, "What's going on?" And he said, "Well, I'm going away. Go here and go there and the third day you have to find somebody to inject you." And I really got quite distressed. The place he suggested was going to be closed the third day, so I had to find somebody myself. So we wound up in the emergency room of his hospital.

The testing and treatment of infertility often involves intricate timing. The doctors or their assistants must schedule postcoital tests, endometrial biopsies, ultrasound evaluation, and artificial insemination according to the woman's ovulation, not the doctor's convenience. This is another good reason to choose a doctor whose practice is entirely or mostly infertility. Obstetricians are frequently called away from the office for deliveries or emergency surgeries.

One time I was supposed to have this insemination (AIH) and my husband couldn't go, so I went alone. Dr. K. didn't show up—the door was locked. I called the service and they said he had an emergency delivery. That really shattered me; I thought I was going to throw myself in front of a bus. It was humiliating and devastating—here I was with my husband's sperm in one hand and this horrible contraption called an azospermia cup in the other. I had a tremendous feeling of helplessness. Here I was, and I was sure I was ovulating. The chart was perfect, and there was nothing I could do.

This woman's story illustrates why it's better to see a fertility specialist than an ob-gyn who delivers many babies. Would you want to miss a chance to get pregnant because another woman is having a baby during your appointment time?

THE FELDMANS

Lisa and Eric were distraught about their fertility problem. They had hoped there was an easy medical explanation for Eric's problem, such as a varicocele, but Eric's doctor was unable to find a specific cause. So he decided to have Eric try HCG (human chorionic gonadotropin), a hormone commonly used to treat female infertility, and occasionally used experimentally to treat male infertility. Eric would have to have two shots of HCG a week for ten weeks and was told that if it worked, they could expect results in three to six months. His urologist, Dr. B., was very optimistic; he gave them a better than good chance of achieving pregnancy. He referred Lisa to a top fertility specialist, Dr. W. Lisa and Eric went together to the first appointment.

LISA: Eric was not with me in the examining room. I was lying on the examining table with my feet in the stirrups feeling nervous and vulnerable, and I said, "Doctor, is everything going to be all right?" And he said, "Listen, Lisa, I don't give it much of a shot." I was crushed.

ERIC: Lisa and I walked out and I'll never forget it. I said to her, "Great news, you're healthy. Dr. W. said to me, 'You can plant any seed in that.' And Lisa looked surprised and said, "But he just told me he doesn't give us much hope." From that point on I don't remember what was said. I was completely devastated. And from that moment on I always heard Dr. W.'s words in the back of my mind. After all, he had the reputation of being the best.

The first time I went to see my urologist, Dr. B., he was my friend. We were buddies and colleagues, and we were going to do everything we could to help me get Lisa pregnant. That's when he first mentioned the HCG shots. I asked about side effects, and he said there were none. I also asked some of my colleagues about the drug, and they assured me there was nothing to worry about.

LISA: Dr. B. said to me, "He may chase you around the bedroom a little bit more." That never happened.

ERIC: The only side effect I had, which he never told me about, was that my breasts got larger and were very sore. I grew breasts, and nobody ever told me that could happen!

After three months I had to go for another semen analysis. It was a cold day and I was sitting on the toilet seat with a nudie magazine, and I felt like I couldn't do it. It was eight-thirty in the morning and I had to get to work; I couldn't just come on demand. It was very dehumanizing—I felt so bad being in there. Lisa was still sleeping and I thought of waking her to help me, but I was finally able to do it. Then I had to bring the sperm sample to the doctor's office and deal with his horrible receptionist.

Here I was sitting in the waiting room with a little brown paper bag. The receptionist pulls the jar out of the bag and holds it up to the light—in front of a room full of people. Here I was trying to be very subtle. It was very important to me—it was my whole life. I just wanted to pick her up and really hurt her. She shouldn't have been in that job because she didn't take in the possibility that men have feelings, that some men are sensitive.

When I made the call to get the results I was terrified and totally confused. I was hoping that what my doctor said was right and that Lisa's doctor was wrong. I made the call from my office, and it was like finding out whether your cancer test was positive. And he treated it like a baseball game! "You can't hit a home run, but that doesn't mean you're out. There's no real change. Keep on hanging in, but I think you should discuss it with Dr. W."

I couldn't believe the change in him. He had been so friendly before, and now he was very aloof. And he had absolutely no questions about how I was feeling. I was devastated. I wanted to write him a letter saying, "People dream their whole lives about having children—it's not just the women—and now you're telling me I'm snuffed out, and you're making a joke of it!" It was so painful. Thank God I had therapy—that helped a lot—and I had Lisa. I called her at her office to give her the bad news.

I was supposed to go back for a six-month checkup but I never did, because I couldn't stand to be humiliated again—giving a sample again. I haven't heard from Dr. B. since. He has no idea what's happening to me, and I don't think he gives a damn.

HOW IMPORTANT IS IT
THAT YOU LIKE YOUR DOCTOR?

It's unfortunate that insensitive doctors like Dr. B. are treating such an emotionally charged disorder as infertility. But even the most sensitive doctors often have a hard time telling a couple that there is no hope. And rather than getting angry at their fate, the couple may react by getting angry at the doctor.

A physician's competence is probably the most important factor to consider when trying to achieve pregnancy, but that doesn't mean you have to be treated by a competent egomaniac. If you absolutely can't stand a doctor, the doctor-patient relationship is bound to suffer, which can surely affect your medical care. And remember, it's not always the doctor's fault—patients can have obnoxious personalities too. According to John Stangel, M.D., a fertility specialist and author of *Fertility and Conception: An Essential Guide for Childless Couples* (New American Library, 1979), choosing a doctor is somewhat akin to choosing a friend.

> The patient's choice of a doctor should be based not only on academic credentials and clinical expertise, but also on ease of communication. Both the doctor and the patient should feel at ease with each other.

Some patients try to disregard a doctor's personality, but unless some rapport exists, the doctor-patient relationship is likely to suffer.

> Dr. N. seemed to know what he was doing, but I couldn't stand his personality. I would grit my teeth and say, All right now, this isn't a personality test. At one point I asked him a question and didn't care for his answer. And I told him that I found him distant and very difficult to get answers from, which made me feel better, but didn't change him. So I took a kind of sneaky way out—I simply stopped going, which is what I think most people would do. So what are you going to do? I mean, if you tell him his personality doesn't jive with yours, what difference is that going to make?

Most patients find it extremely difficult to confront a doctor over medical issues, let alone personality issues. However, if enough patients complain to a doctor about his personality, it may ultimately make a difference. Perhaps you can suggest that he work with an infertility counselor, who can pay special attention to your emotional needs (see chapter 6).

When looking for an infertility specialist, it may pay to interview several before you make your decision. You can, for medical and insurance purposes, consider this a second opinion and have two evaluations of your medical condition. Then you can take each doctor's personality into account as well as their medical skills, as did one woman trying to decide between two doctors; she had left her first doctor because she found him insensitive to her emotional needs.

Dr. P. spent just an unbelievable amount of time with me, and he was very kind. He listened to me go on, with nurses banging on the door telling him he had patients waiting. He waited for me to end the interview. Then I went to see Dr. Z. He was very businesslike, and I was very impressed with his technical abilities. But at that point, after my treatment with my first doctor, I felt I really needed someone who was sensitive, and Dr. P. had the edge on Dr. Z. in that area.

Of course, you have to be careful not to sacrifice technical skills just for the sake of a good personality. Ideally, that combination can be found in the same person.

I was impressed with my doctor because I believed he knew what he was talking about, and he was much more rational and scientific than anybody I'd seen up to that point. But also he was in tune with the whole emotional side of it. Despite being department chairman, he was the easiest person to reach of all the doctors that I had seen. He was very available and very supportive.

According to Miriam Mazor, M.D., clinical professor in psychiatry at Harvard Medical School:

The myth of the best or "top" doctor is unrealistic. In a large medical center there are usually choices of equally competent doctors with different styles. Some patients find one doctor supportive, while others may find him or her patronizing. Some patients prefer an aggressive "go for it" approach, while others prefer a slower and more cautious pace. What is important is the "fit" between doctor and patient.

SHOULD YOU SWITCH DOCTORS?

If you do feel that your present physician is not competent in the field of infertility, you should absolutely find a new doctor. But if you just can't stand him, what should you do? Says Dr. Stangel, "Even if a doctor has the highest credentials, there are times when the chemistry between the doctor and patient does not work out; then it's reasonable to switch doctors." Unless you live in an area where there is only one fertility specialist, your doctor is not the only one who can help you. If you're unhappy with him or her, start looking elsewhere for a new doctor.

I hated my doctor but hadn't considered changing; I hadn't met anybody else who was infertile, and I really didn't know what alternatives existed. I just felt like it was my craziness that I couldn't stand the man. Then I spoke to a woman who had just adopted privately. She asked me about my doctor. I started describing him. She said, "I don't mean to intrude, but . . ." She not only validated my feelings that this was a miserable way to be treated by a doctor, but also that just because I was infertile didn't mean that I should have a bastard for a doctor.

Talking to other men and women with fertility problems is a good way of helping you determine whether you're in the best hands medically. It is also an excellent source of referral for finding a fertility specialist. Again, don't just take someone's suggestion at face value without doing some further checking with RESOLVE, The American Fertility Society, or the other organizations mentioned earlier in this chapter. Just because someone you meet becomes pregnant while using a certain doctor doesn't mean that her doctor will be the right one for you.

Inadequate training in infertility, suspected medical incompetence, or an irritating personality are not the only valid reasons for switching doctors. If you or your doctor feel that there is nothing more he can do for you, it is time to seek another opinion.

After I had been using condoms and taking steroids for a sperm antibody problem, my doctor said to me, "If you don't get pregnant after the year on condoms and steroids, then you'll never get pregnant. So if you're not pregnant in two or three months, there's nothing to be done—you'll have to adopt." At which point I switched doctors. He was very nice, but he had nothing else to offer.

Some people, not necessarily unreasonably, believe that if they have not gotten pregnant with a certain doctor after a certain period of time trying, it's time to switch. This may make sense especially if the woman is in her thirties; she may not want to spend too much time with any one doctor. This was the case with one woman in her midthirties who was herself a physician.

I had a long succession of gynecologists. As a doctor, I always had excellent access to doctors, and I could switch doctors at my whim, almost. I'd give each doctor about a year and then switch doctors.

On the other hand, doctors can't make much headway with a particular patient's problem overnight. A doctor should be given enough time to try various treatments and evaluate their results. Dr. Stangel advises, "As long as you feel your treatment is moving along, then you can stay with your doctor even if it seems to be taking a long time. But if you feel you are treading water, it's time to move on."

Dr. Stangel also recommends that patients sit down with their doctors and review or reevaluate their medical therapy every three or four months. Says Dr. Stangel, "Medical therapy is a cooperative venture. The couple should have a feeling of active, not passive, participation in their own treatment." If your doctor is too busy during your regular appointment time to discuss your case with you, make an appointment just to talk to him. It will be worth the cost to get a good, honest evaluation of your situation and help you anticipate what the doctor has in store for you six to twelve months down the road if you still aren't pregnant. If your doctor refuses to have a conference with you, it's definitely time to find someone who is more accommodating.

Many couples find it exceedingly difficult to switch doctors even when they know their doctor is not right for them. They may feel a sense of loyalty, fear of hurting their doctor's feelings, fear of dealing with a new doctor, fear of the unknown, or a combination of all the above. As RESOLVE's president, Beverly Freeman, explains:

> It's very hard for people to switch doctors even if they're having a terrible time with their current doctor. They have all kinds of reservations about it that run the gamut from the inconvenience involved in making the change to being afraid to confront the doctor about their need for a second opinion. Second opinions are common, and if your doctor demonstrates any resistance, you probably shouldn't be with him in the first place.

American Fertility Society president Dr. Wallach gives the following advice about switching doctors and getting a second opinion:

> A patient should change physicians any time she feels uncomfortable in her association with a physician. [And] it is important for any patient to feel free and comfortable to receive a second opinion. If her physician resists having a second opinion, it usually indicates a lack of self-confidence.

HOW TO SWITCH DOCTORS PAINLESSLY

Even when someone makes the decision to switch doctors, he or she often goes through terrible angst about making that final break. According to Beverly Freeman,

> . . . it's because of the special bond between a patient and a doctor, especially in infertility, because the doctors are the symbols of hope. And you wonder if you are going to step backward in some fashion by leaving and starting again. I think it's important to remember you may be gaining lots of time, and it may be the best choice you ever made.

Dr. Stangel suggests that you merely call or write the doctor a short note saying something like the following:

Dear Dr. _____,
    Please send a copy of my medical records to Dr. _____, (address).

Thank you for your attention and courtesy over the past few years (months).

Sincerely,

If you are especially afraid of hurting the doctor's feelings, and have been fairly satisfied with the doctor, you might say something such as:

> I find this letter very difficult to write because I've been very pleased with your treatment of me. However, since I still am not pregnant, I would like to have another opinion.

And if the doctor is encouraging you to stop treatment or adopt, and you wish to pursue more medical treatment, Dr. Stangel recommends saying something like the following:

> We find it difficult to accept your diagnosis that we should give up at this point, and we feel obligated to leave no stone unturned. So we will be continuing treatment with Dr. _____. We're deeply appreciative of all you've done for us up to this point.

Doctors should not and probably will not be offended by such letters. Don't forget, you are only one of perhaps hundreds of patients your doctor sees. But he is the only one you see—so, to put it bluntly, he means a lot more to you than you do to him. Says Dr. Stangel:

> I strongly feel patients are in charge of their own destiny. If someone doesn't like the way I put on my hat or my medical treatment, and wants to try something or someone else, I'm not offended.

If you are planning to write to the doctor to complain about his treatment of you, there are no special guidelines to follow except that you should, in a straightforward manner, describe in detail what it is that you are upset about. And if you have any helpful suggestions, by all means make them—they may benefit his other patients. Of course, there's no telling what his reaction will be, but if you are displeased with him it probably makes no difference. There will be no further doctor-patient relationship to worry about, and you certainly won't be sending your friends to him for treatment!

THE SPANELLIS

Sue was very upset with the medical treatment she had been receiving and was very disappointed in her doctor. She believed she and Anthony had wasted two years without finding out a thing about the cause of their infertility. She was ready to switch doctors but had difficulty making the final break. Also, Anthony was against changing doctors.

ANTHONY: I was very hesitant to switch. I felt we should stick with Dr. T. because she came highly recommended and because she was a woman. And I felt like we'd be starting over again.

SUE: She told us to try on our own for a few more months and then call her. We were still not sure of our judgment on this, so we did as she suggested. Nothing happened, so I telephoned her. She didn't return my call. Then I called again and she was very annoyed—she was actually angry that I had called! I said, "Well, you told me to call after a few months," and she said by a few months she meant six months. Here I was, thirty-seven years old and still not pregnant!

I kept trying to press her to give her medical opinion about what to do next and whether we should do more inseminations. She said she didn't think more inseminations made sense and then said, "I think you're being too emotional about this." I said, "Well, I've been trying to get pregnant for two years and nothing has worked," and she said, "What do you expect with a subfertile husband!" I don't even know what I said at that point. I was at work. I hung up the phone, closed the door to my office, and put my head down on my desk and cried. That's when I knew I wasn't going back to her.

ANTHONY: When Sue told me what happened, I said, "Now what the hell are we going to do?" I really didn't know what to do.

SUE: I knew by then we needed a fertility specialist. I looked in the Yellow Pages and found a fertility clinic. I made an appointment but didn't tell Dr. T., because we still weren't positive we had done the right thing.

ANTHONY: When we went in for our appointment, they took a thorough history and did some simple lab tests that we hadn't had done before.

SUE: They did more that first day that was constructive than Dr. T. had done in two years! We were there the whole morning. And then we met the doctor we were assigned to, Dr. P. We liked him immediately. He seemed competent and understanding. And he answered all our questions. He seemed surprised that Dr. T. hadn't done any tests. He said, "She didn't do a postcoital? She didn't do any tests? She just did a laparoscopy?" When we left the clinic, we turned to each other and said. "We're doing the right thing!"

Dr. P. put me on Clomid. I was on it for six months and no pregnancy. He then suggested we try Pergonal. Initially the thought of taking Pergonal was an up, because we were trying something new.

ANTHONY: I thought, Wow, Pergonal, the heavy artillery, the wonder drug, the miracle drug, all the quintuplets you read about. I thought, This is top of the line—we can't miss.

SUE: I saw it as the end of the line, because we had no particular diagnosis; Anthony's sperm count was still good. It was a bit depressing and scary because it seemed so complicated—all the shots and blood tests. I talked it over with my doctor and then with Anthony. I told him all the pros and cons and said, "But we know we're going to do it, don't we?" I also told him that the doctor said it usually costs at least $800 to $900 per month including all the blood tests and sonograms. He agreed we should try it. Our first cycle was $1800! We had sperm washings and inseminations and I had a long cycle that month, so that added to the cost. [Inseminations and sperm washings cost about $125 to $200 per insemination.]

ANTHONY: We had double insurance coverage, so luckily all of it was covered.

HOW TO GET REIMBURSED
BY YOUR INSURANCE COMPANY

While childlessness is a *social* condition, infertility is a symptom that something is *physically* wrong with the reproductive system. It is therefore a medical condition, for which every patient who has medical insurance is entitled to coverage. Unfortunately, not all insurance companies see it that way. And to make matters worse, not all doctors care whether their patients get reimbursed for their services, as long as their bills are paid.

Throughout the United States, there are uniform diagnostic codes and procedures for filling out health insurance forms, and your doctor and his staff should be aware of what they are so you can be reimbursed. According to RESOLVE's Beverly Freeman, "Companies will reject a claim that says 'infertility treatment' because it doesn't fit into a certain code. So the claim should not say 'infertility' on it." However, she points out, there are many standard procedures that—when viewed in themselves and not as part of an infertility treatment—are perfectly appropriate for insurance coding and billing. "All the codes are encompassing enough," she writes, "that they permit you to classify almost any infertility treatment into the appropriate category." For example, there may not be a code for T-*Mycoplasma* testing, but there will be a code for testing for infections. Says Ms. Freeman, "If the doctor or his bookkeeper does not know how to file claims so he patient is reimbursed, and the doctor can't rectify that situation, the patient should switch doctors. That commonly happens when the doctor does not do a lot of infertility work. Anyone who is in the business has an incentive to make sure his patients are covered."

Ms. Freeman also points out that a lot of claims have to be filed by patients, and they should learn how to fill out the forms or should contact their benefits office for help. Unfortunately, this usually involves the benefits officer learning about the patient's fertility problem; many people may not want their employers to find out they are trying to conceive, much less having problems doing so. Each couple has to weigh the financial benefits of being reimbursed against the risk of having their boss discover that they have a fertility problem.

THE FELDMANS

After Lisa and Eric got over the initial shock of finding out the HCG shots hadn't improved Eric's sperm, they went back to see Lisa's doctor, Dr. W., to see if anything could be done—and to ascertain whether their case was indeed hopeless.

LISA: Dr. W. suggested that we try artificial insemination with Eric's sperm [AIH]. He said he wanted to give it a shot before looking at other options.

ERIC: I had another semen analysis, this time using Dr. W.'s lab so I wouldn't have to deal with my urologist again. When Dr. W. looked at the sperm under the microscope he said, "That's not so bad." So here was someone else giving me another inkling of a possibility that I was going to be able to father a child.

LISA: He did the first insemination, which was really no big deal. Eric was with me in the room. Then forty-eight hours later, on a Saturday, he scheduled another insemination. He was going to be away so he arranged for his nurse, who is lovely, to do it.

ERIC: When Lisa and I went to the office that Saturday, we were feeling quite optimistic. But when the nurse looked at the semen under the microscope, there was hardly anything there—there were virtually no sperm. I was distraught and said, "Why bother doing the insemination? Let's go home." But the nurse insisted that we do it. She said, "All you need is one."

THE COOPERS

Mai Li's doctor, Dr. S., had removed as many of the lesions caused by the endometriosis as he could during Mai Li's laparoscopy. He then gave them two options. They could try to get pregnant on their own, or Mai Li could take danazol (Danocrine), a drug routinely used to treat endometriosis. It produces a temporary cessation of ovulation, causing the endometriosis lesions to shrink and preventing new ones from growing. He explained that she would have to take the drug for at least six months and that there might be some unpleasant side effects such as weight gain, acne, and possibly facial hair growth. Also, she would not menstruate or ovulate for six months, which meant she could not possibly get pregnant for those six months. The couple chose the first option.

MAI LI: We tried to get pregnant for six months after the surgery and nothing happened. Dr. S. again recommended danazol—he called it the final card up his sleeve. I took danazol for six months and did in fact gain ten pounds, but had none of the other side effects.

After six months on danazol and another six months trying to get pregnant without success, I was very upset and very discouraged. Dr. S. said it was time to have a second-look laparoscopy. But my feeling at that point was that Dr. S. had his chance, now someone else was going to get a chance. By then I had joined RESOLVE and had been hearing about other specialists in the area I hadn't heard about before. One of them was Dr. E. Everybody was raving about him, so I figured why not. I told Dr. S. that before I had surgery again, I wanted a second opinion. I was a little bit anxious about telling him because of the way the doctor-patient relationship is set up, but his reaction was, "OK, fine. I can recommend some people." I mentioned Dr. E. and his response was, "He's excellent."

ROY: I also thought it was a good idea to get a second opinion. As much as I liked Dr. S., he seemed to have nothing else to offer. I remember being in Dr. S.'s office after the six months on danazol, and he was discouraged—his attitude had become pessimistic and depressing. He said, "I don't like this; it's not good. If Mai Li hasn't gotten pregnant after the danazol, I'm not optimistic." I remember the walk downtown after that appointment with Dr. S. It was a gray day, just about to drizzle. I don't remember feeling so depressed. I would start to say something and just sigh—I was practically in tears. I thought, It's over. All the optimism, all the struggling, all the attempts, all the work, all the sex on schedule, all the doctor's visits, the surgery, the pain, the decision making—and it was all a waste.

CHAPTER 3

The infertility puts a lot of pressure on him. He brings me flowers. He takes me out to dinner. He buys me pretty things. He's an inordinately loving and supportive husband. He's a super husband. But the one thing I want most, he can't give me.

THE INFERTILE MARRIAGE

THE SPANELLIS

Sue was now taking Pergonal, a potent fertility drug that requires one injection a day for about five to ten days prior to ovulation at midcycle. Although the doctor suggested that Anthony give her the shots, Anthony couldn't trust himself to do it, so the doctor taught Sue how to self-administer the shots.

> SUE: When I got to the point of actually injecting myself, I just couldn't do it. I was in the bedroom and stood there and stood there and would prick myself a little and then chicken out. I finally came out into the living room and said, "Don't you think you could possibly do this? I really can't do it myself." And he said he would.
>
> ANTHONY: It took me a half hour of pacing back and forth to work up the nerve, but I was finally able to do it.

SUE: It really helped me to have him give me those injections, because it involved him more. Even though he had had surgery for varicoceles, that had been several years before. Most of the time I tended to feel that I was carrying the whole burden in terms of trying to get pregnant—that all the things were being done to my body, and that I was the one who had to keep running to the doctor's office. He didn't have to go to doctors' offices or have a lot of invasive procedures, but at least he was giving me injections. It made me feel he was more involved in the process.

Both Anthony and Sue were optimistic about the Pergonal. And during the second cycle, they saw two follicles on the sonogram—an indication that Sue would probably ovulate two eggs.

SUE: I thought, Wow! Twins! It was hard not to feel encouraged—you see those two little things on the sonogram. And then two weeks later, I got my period.

ANTHONY: And it kept on coming with really depressing regularity for months. That was the only thing that was predictable about the whole process.

SUE: The doctor could see that it was very emotionally difficult for us and was very sensitive to our feelings. This doctor could always take time to talk, even if he had a waiting room full of patients.

After I was on Pergonal for seven months, we decided we needed a break. We had not had a break from my trying to get pregnant for three and a half years. So we told Dr. P. we wanted to take a break, but for only one month, because I was concerned about my age—I was almost thirty-nine. We also told him we were going to start exploring adoption. One reason was that we felt the infertility was having a detrimental effect on our relationship.

We started to have a lot of arguments, but not directly related to infertility. The biggest one was during our worst time in terms of the infertility. We had had seven frustrating cycles on Pergonal. I was angry about everything. By that time I'd gone through so much in terms of medical procedures, and so much emotionally. And one day I came home with a lot of complaints about Anthony and said to him that rather than telling his family we were seriously considering adopting, we should tell them that we were getting a divorce—that I really thought we had serious problems in our marriage.

ANTHONY: I really blew my top; I just let her have it. I told her, "You'll never find another husband like me, you're pretty damn lucky to have someone like me for a husband, and I don't know what the hell you're getting so angry about." Because I really didn't know.

SUE: Then he told me all the reasons he thought he was a good husband, and I had to agree with all of them! Sort of meekly, apologizing. I think we ended up realizing that the problems that we really had were the problems with infertility.

ANTHONY: The infertility was not something we could just surround and isolate and leave alone. It just permeated our entire life. It would not leave us alone.

SUE: Part of what was playing into my anger and frustration was frustration about our sexual relationship. I don't think either of us was enjoying sex during that time.

ANTHONY: Because there was that same thing in the back of our minds—getting pregnant! We hated to have to schedule sex around pregnancy all the time. I always felt like I had to save myself for the right moment.

SUE: There had not been any time when we had had unscheduled sex when I hadn't wondered beforehand whether it would be detrimental to my getting pregnant because we might use up the good sperm. I tended always to be the one saying, "I don't think this would be a good time to have sex; it's too close to when I'll ovulate."

ANTHONY: I think it's a tribute to us that we stuck together. For one thing, we never really blamed each other for our infertility problems—it wasn't something we caused. It was something we were both working very hard to overcome. This is a trial we were going through. And we would survive it, we would beat it.

Regardless of who has the problem, infertility is a couples' problem. It's a problem that involves every aspect of those it

touches: self-image, self-esteem, and sexuality. When one partner fails, the other fails. For some, it's the first time they have
failed at anything so major. And with failure comes guilt, blame,
resentment, depression, shame, and anger.

ANGER

Like Anthony and Sue, many couples react to infertility with
generalized anger.

It made us both angry that Mary wasn't getting pregnant. She
was getting hurt, worried, and depressed. I was just plain
angry. You don't even know who or what you're angry at. It
seemed like my life was screwed up and I was angry at myself
or Mary or the doctor or whatever, and it spilled over into
everything.

And sometimes the anger is expressed indirectly by saying
hurtful things.

There were conversations where my husband would say the
worst that he could say, which was, "Gee, I wanted to see you
all pregnant with your breasts full of milk and taste the milk."
He is Swedish and would talk about how we would never
have a kid with Swedish blood because I was infertile.

If they don't drive a couple apart, hurtful, hostile remarks
may bring things to a head and can help a couple reevaluate
their situations.

We had one very traumatic fight a few months ago after we
had a husband insemination. I said to him, "We never should
have gotten married." And he said to me, "Well, I hope you're
not pregnant, because if you are, then we can't get divorced."
I said, "I don't care, you do whatever you want. But if I'm
pregnant, I'm having this baby whether we're married or not.
I can support this baby and I can take care of it." And he just
burst into tears. He totally fell apart. And he said, "You know
I love you and want a baby more than anything." And that
was sort of a turning point.

Infertility is a major life crisis for both spouses, and it's virtually impossible for any marriage to remain unscathed by it. Most couples have their ups and downs, but the infertile couple has these with unrelenting frequency, usually following the ups and downs of the temperature chart.

Husbands and wives react differently to infertility. Even if the husband is the one with the fertility problem, it is the wife who must monitor her body for signs of ovulation and pregnancy. Diagnostic tests for women are often complex, frightening, and painful. Diagnostic tests for men are less invasive and painful, given that the most common test for the man—semen analysis—involves masturbation. Some men may find producing a semen sample emotionally difficult, but it is certainly not physically painful! As one woman graphically and angrily put it, "I get biopsied, dye shot in my tubes, operated upon, not to mention internal exams—and I'm not even sick! And all he has to do is jerk off, lucky bastard!"

CONFLICTS

Wives tend to be not only physically more involved in the infertility, but emotionally as well. And this often leads to conflicts or arguments.

Both my husband and I had fertility problems. I can't say that he wasn't cooperating, but in a very subtle way he wasn't involved. He was paying the bills when they came every month, but it was my project really. So we would get into these picayune arguments. For example, my husband likes to take hot showers, and that's supposed to be harmful to sperm. I would say, "I really don't think you should be taking hot showers. *I* would suffocate in the bathroom with that kind of heat." And of course he would get angry.

Many husbands, however, are often more involved than their wives realize—they just have more difficulty expressing it, both emotionally and verbally.

I felt that Sam wasn't as concerned about the infertility as I was. I was doing most of the work: I was the one who had to go to the doctor, and I was the one who had to get the injections, and I was the one who had to make the appointments and call the doctor and get the lab results. And I was the one who kept bringing it up for discussion, like when should we think about adoption? Or when should I change doctors? Or should I have the laparoscopy? He wouldn't spontaneously bring it up until about six months ago when he had just come back from a friend's wedding in his home town. Most of his old friends were married with two-point-four children. He came home and said he'd never seen so many beautiful kids. His first day back, we were getting ready to go out to dinner and I got my period. The next night at the dinner table, after I got through complaining how awful my life was, he said to me, "You know, last night when you told me that you'd gotten your period, I felt like you stabbed me. I realize that even though you accuse me of not being concerned about the infertility, I really am. In fact I'm so concerned about it I can't even deal with it—it's really hard on me." And we both started crying.

Usually the wife wants to talk about infertility more than her husband does, and this can create tension in the marriage; many wives believe their husbands' lack of interest in discussing the issue means a lack of involvement. Whether this is true or not, it can lead to tension and arguments. Wives often get angry at their husbands for not wanting to discuss infertility. Sometimes they have to literally corner their husbands to get them to discuss the issue.

Phil doesn't like to discuss these things. So I follow him to the bathroom when he soaks his back. I found that was the best place to have discussions—either on a very long trip when we're in the car for eight hours, or when he has to soak his back.

And many husbands get angry at their wives for constantly bringing up the subject, especially in front of other people.

In the beginning, when I used to talk about our fertility problem with others, my husband couldn't stand it. He would get furious. Now it doesn't bother him so much. He found it very embarrassing; I guess he felt emasculated. He didn't want anybody to think it was his fault or his problem. I guess he would rather have people assume that if we didn't have children, it was because we didn't want children, that we had great careers without children.

SOLUTIONS

It's unrealistic to assume that both spouses will want to discuss infertility to the same extent or with the same intensity, explained Kate Gorman, D.S.W., a psychotherapist who specializes in treating infertile couples. "The important thing to remember is to respect each other's sensitivities about the issue," advises Dr. Gorman. "Each person has the right to deal with infertility in his or her own way."

If you feel a great need to discuss infertility and your spouse doesn't, you may have friends who also have fertility problems with whom you can talk. If not, perhaps you should look into finding a support group, such as RESOLVE, made up of others with similar problems. Support groups for couples are especially helpful in getting the less-involved spouse more involved. (see chapter 6).

Another way of getting your spouse more involved is to suggest he or she read books about infertility; they can act as catalysts for discussion. Of course, it's not easy to get a person to read who doesn't want to.

Jack is very supportive, but sometimes I think he doesn't want to talk about it enough. I've practically had to threaten to kill him if he didn't read the fertility book I bought. I told him again last night, "I'm going to kill you if you haven't read the book by tonight! And I'm going to give you a quiz!" But what I failed to remember is that he has to do it when he wants to and when his mind is receptive to it. And he seems to think he's more receptive to it on the subway than at home. So if he wants to sit on the subway and read a book on infertility and have his friends or whoever he might happen to meet see him reading the book, that's cool.

There are times when you will have to discuss your fertility problem with your spouse, for example when you must make important decisions about medical treatment or adoption. If your spouse refuses at that point to get involved, then perhaps it would be best for you to seek help from a marriage counselor.

Working together toward a common goal is perhaps the most productive thing a couple can do, both for their fertility problem and for their marriage. Dr. Gorman says one way of sharing the load is to involve your spouse in the medical process, for example, by going to doctors' appointments with your spouse whenever possible. In that way, you can provide emotional support while receiving medical information about your problem. Says Dr. Gorman, "It feels more like a couple's effort than an individual effort if you at least attempt to go to all the tests and treatments that are in any way stressful or painful." Even being there to sit in the waiting room can help.

EMPATHY

It often helps a marriage if each spouse can understand what the other is going through—the pain, the humiliation, and the frustration that so often accompany infertility.

My husband went through a job experience which is in many ways for a man analogous to trying to have a baby for a woman. He interviewed for a job that he very, very much wanted. They told him he was one of the finalists, but he's never been called for a reinterview, so he doesn't know if he really is or isn't still in the running. After the first interview, which went very well, he was talking about how in about two weeks he'd know whether he was going to get a second interview. Those two weeks were like the second half of my menstrual cycle—every day he thought about it all the time. He fantasized about it. He went over every word of that interview the way I would go over my temperature chart to see if I made it. And each day that he didn't get a call he would say, "Well, you know, it's Thanksgiving week"—the same kind of things that I would think. And toward the end of that time he said to me, "You know, I don't want to fantasize about it in case I'm disappointed." And I said, "Listen, I can tell you from experience that whether you fantasize about it or not, you're going to be disappointed if you don't get it. And as long as you keep your fantasy and reality straight, enjoy the fantasy." I said it was just like infertility, and—I can't describe what his face looked like. He just looked horrified and he said, "You mean that's what it's been like for you?"

HAVING FUN

Each couple has to work out for themselves what might help them survive this trying period in their marriage. It may help to remember that there are other dimensions to your marriage that can and should be cultivated. Said one man, "It helps to keep in mind that you still have all the fun of marriage available to you that you had before you discovered this problem." Dr. Gorman, in fact, recommends that you make having fun with your spouse a priority in your marriage, even if you have to work at it.

We weren't having much fun for a long time. Our New Year's resolution for three years in a row has been—we have to have more fun. We have to do recreational things together. We're getting too caught up in just work, housework, and trying to get pregnant. So we've been working at having more fun— going skiing, going to the movies, and just going out more.

THE FELDMANS

Lisa and Eric had a lot of stress in their marriage. Lisa's father was dying, and they had a serious fertility problem. Lisa's desire for a child became more intense because she knew her father, to whom she was very close, was not going to live much longer. She wanted him to be a grandfather, or at least have a child to name after him if he died. Soon after Eric found that the HCG shots he had taken had not worked, Lisa's father died. Lisa was distraught; she had lost her father at the same time she discovered her husband could not father the child she so desperately hoped for.

LISA: The only thing I had that I felt was good in my life was our marriage; luckily, we were getting along better than we ever had before. From the moment we got Eric's diagnosis, we got closer and tighter than I ever imagined we would get.

ERIC: When we got married, we had a tendency to split and go in different directions when we had a conflict. But our marriage was coming together, especially after Lisa's dad had died. So when we had disagreements about what to do about the infertility, we talked about it and worked it out.

LISA: We never fought about it; in fact, it brought us closer together. We had a common goal, and we worked together. And we never blamed each other for the problem.

ERIC: The one thing I always tried to do when I got really frustrated and angry about our fertility problem was not to take it out on Lisa and become moody. You start to become a whiner, you want to be held, you want to be caressed, you just want to be cared for because you're so damn miserable.

LISA: We held each other a lot, but we became less sexual.

ERIC: They told me when I took the medication [HCG] that it would increase my sexual activity, but that never happened. In fact, things got worse. I guess I was insecure. We had always had a very good sex life up until then, but it changed at that point. Although I never really had any trouble performing, I was worried about it. It became such a head trip that I needed a vacation from sex—I wanted to be left alone. I couldn't stand it. Sex became very confusing and very unreal. I know it was all related to that diagnosis of, "Hey, mister, you've only got X amount of sperm and not much motility, so we'll call you subfertile." Sex really changed for me from that point on.

LISA: When he wasn't interested in sex, I didn't take it personally; I felt sorry for him. I felt bad—I knew that he was going through hell, and there was nothing I could do. I didn't even trust myself to say the right thing.

I lost intere t in sex, too. I forgot about it. I'd start reading in bed at night. It wouldn't have dawned on me to initiate sex for pleasure. We were lucky; it was convenient that we both didn't give a damn about sex. When he wasn't interested, it took a big weight off me because I wasn't all that interested.

But it wasn't painful not having sex, it wasn't terrible or uncomfortable.

ERIC: Lisa's lack of interest was predicated on the fact that I was going through craziness, and my lack of interest was based on whether I was macho. As much as I tried to deny it, it was there. I was like that. All the input was there from all those years. I kept having visions of eunuchs—I went through all that shit.

Lisa helped me a lot by being very supportive and loving. She also helped me a lot by saying, "Your thyroid is bad, you take your thyroid pills. Your sperm count is low, you take this medicine." It really made sense to me, because it had nothing to do with something I could control. It wasn't my fault I had a thyroid problem, and it wasn't my fault that there was something wrong with my sperm. It was not me, but it became me for a while.

THE SEXUAL RELATIONSHIP

The association between fertility and virility is very strong, especially in men's minds. When fertility is impaired, a man's sense of his virility also often becomes impaired. This can easily lead to sexual problems, or fears of sexual inadequacy, as it did for Eric.

Scheduled Sex

A couple's sex life, not surprisingly, is perhaps the area most dramatically affected by infertility. It is no longer just the husband and wife in bed. The thermometer and doctor's orders are ever-present, dictating when the couple should or should not have sexual intercourse.

When I was on Pergonal, I would call my doctor when my temperature was about to go down and she would say, "OK, have intercourse tonight, tomorrow, and the next day." Well, you can't perform that way. It's horrendous. You feel like animals, not human beings. So it has made us the best of friends and very lousy sex partners.

Scheduled sex cannot help but affect a couple's sex life—the couple are no longer involved in making love, but in making babies.

You're forced to have sex to try and impregnate your wife, and then it gets related to specific times of the month and it becomes a chore—sometimes it's a pleasant chore and sometimes it's not. Instead of being something you think of that you spontaneously turn to for warmth and pleasure and fun, it becomes associated with duty. Certainly the recreational aspects become minimal and the procreational aspects become huge, because you're failing to procreate—and that's not so great.

Scheduled sex very commonly leads to lack of sexual interest, impotence, frigidity, and arguments. And if the couple doesn't have a terrific sex life to begin with, the problems can grow and become a threat to their relationship.

Sex was never a really strong suit for us. We get along in so many other ways, and infertility has attacked the weakest part of the marriage, which is the sexual part. And so, needless to say, it has really wreaked havoc. My husband is extremely loving and affectionate and supportive. But he's not a particularly sexual man. Being called upon to perform just puts another millstone around his neck. And I feel like I'm demanding sexual performance, which makes me feel totally inhibited. It's really lousy—I mean, I really don't like sex any more. It's not any fun any more.

I think Chris probably knows that I'm lying there thinking, "Just deposit the sperm and leave," which is essentially all I'm interested in. I'm not interested in sex any more. I'm interested in conception. I wish it weren't so, but that's the way it really is. If I could take a little pill in the morning instead of having sex, I would rather do that—that would be wonderful.

The lack of sexual interest or the inability to perform on schedule can be misinterpreted as a desire not to have a child.

We were supposed to have sex every other day in midcyle, but there was a problem with that because my husband is not the kind of person who can be put on a schedule like that, and he really rebelled. And I was very angry. I was angry because I didn't understand why if he really wanted to have children, he couldn't do what he was supposed to do. I didn't feel that he gave it the ol' college try.

A lack of sexual interest on the part of one partner can threaten any marriage. But in the infertile marriage, since sex is more equated with babies than with pleasure, the foundations of the marriage may be more easily shaken.

Sometimes I think that maybe if he was more sexually interested . . . You just don't know any more. I think this is just a monumental marital crisis. I have thoughts in my very dark, dark moments that maybe it's just my chemistry with his that's not working out. Maybe I should contact an old boyfriend or something. Not for an affair, not for kicks. But just for this right sperm, in my search for this master sperm that can find its way to this very obviously elusive egg.

Frustration

Sexual problems and frustration can make one spouse wonder if the other really loves him or her, and this can lead to resentment and arguments.

Sex for a couple of years was horrible, just horrible. I thought, Oh well, I really love this guy. But it really makes you question. You know you love him but you really wonder, because you're not getting anything out of sex. Even if I didn't tell Tim it was that time of the month, there was such pressure to make sure we were having intercourse every other night for a few nights in a row—there just wasn't any enjoyment. And I would sometimes just turn over and say, It's not worth it. I would really get upset and accuse him of not loving me.

The frustration is not just sexual. As one woman told me, "Psychologically you connect sex with failure, so you're going through the motions of doing something that time and again has been proven to be clinically unsuccessful, and that's what's so frustrating."

Both kinds of frustration, the sexual frustration and the frustration of failure, inevitably lead to arguments, especially when it's time for scheduled sex.

And then of course there was scheduled sex—that's where the fights get played out the most. Amy would say, "It's tonight," and I would say, "Oh, God, no!" and complain about hating to have to perform on schedule and things like that. So it really had a terrible effect on our sex life. And it spilled over into other areas and made sex a kind of battleground. It becomes, "We have to do it tonight." And I'd say, "I don't want to do it tonight." "Well, you have to do it tonight." "Well, I don't want to—what's the matter with tomorrow night?" "Well, tomorrow night is not the right night." Then if I don't do it on the right night and we don't get pregnant at the end of the month, then of course it's my fault.

Scheduled sex can also involve just the man if he has to produce a semen specimen at a specific time. But that too can lead to arguments and resentment.

The only difficulty we have with sex is getting my husband to masturbate for artificial inseminations—he resents having to masturbate on schedule because that's always in the morning. If it were at night I don't think it would be so much of a problem. The big deal is this jerking off into a jar in the morning when he has to go to work. And I'm late too, and I have to sit there pleading with him when he says, "I'm not going to do it today." He gets angry about having to do it—he says it makes him tenser at work.

Not only is scheduled sex a common occurrence in infertility, but so is scheduled abstention, as one woman sadly discovered.

Our sex life is nonexistent. I think in the last year we had normal sex once. I don't even know what it's like any more. First of all, when I finally got pregnant, the doctor said we should abstain for three months. Then I had a miscarriage and he said abstain for six months! Then we started again and had all these hangups and fears and everything. For a while, things got normal again. But then we started the husband inseminations, and we were told to abstain for several days at a time to build up the sperm count.

Not everyone dislikes scheduled sex. One woman told me, "My husband loves it because he figures we have sex more frequently, and he thinks that's great."

Sexual Solutions

Scheduled sex is a reality for most infertile couples—but it may help to remember that it's only a temporary situation. According to Roselle Shubin, an infertility counselor in New York City, "In order to survive scheduled sex, you should realize that it's not passionate lovemaking, but scientifically determined sexual intercourse." And, advises Ms. Shubin, "you should understand each other's physiological limits, and not interpret them as rejection."

There are things couples can do to survive scheduled sex and even enhance their sex lives at the same time.

Scheduled sex wasn't a problem, because I wouldn't tell Bob it was scheduled sex. I wouldn't say, "Listen, you've got to be home tonight or else." What I would do is use a little seduction.

Every infertile couple has probably been told more times than they'd like to remember to "just relax" or "take a vacation" as if that would get them pregnant. Following this advice won't help them conceive, but it may enhance their sex lives, as it did for these two couples.

For a while my Nick was having trouble having an erection on the night we were supposed to have sex. He realizes it's tension and we try to work around it. We try to go out to dinner or go to a movie and do things just to help us relax. There was a period during which we were turned off by the whole idea of having sex. We made jokes about it. But the only times we really were able to enjoy it was when we went on vacations and did it in exotic and wonderful places.

If you don't have access to exotic places, a change of scenery might help. Ms. Shubin suggests, "Don't do it in the bedroom at night, do it elsewhere, like on the living-room floor in the afternoon." In fact, Barbara Eck Menning, founder of RESOLVE, suggests in her book, *Infertility: A Guide for the Childless Couple* (Prentice Hall, 1977), that both the bedroom and bedtime should be declared "off limits" for having sex—because this "helps break an old and defeated pattern. Also it restores some humor and spontaneity to the situation."

Because most couples with fertility problems cannot help but associate sexual intercourse with pregnancy, Ms. Menning suggests you try other ways to enjoy sex besides intercourse when you're not ovulating, such as oral sex or mutual masturbation— things that in no way can be associated with pregnancy. Non-procreative sex might also be something to consider if you are able to take a break from infertility by taking a month or two off with no temperature charts and no medical treatment—something each couple should try to do at some point if possible.

Of course, if you and your spouse are having sexual problems that you feel cannot be resolved over time, or if you are constantly fighting about sex, then it would make good sense to seek professional help from a qualified sex therapist or marriage counselor (see chapter 6).

THE COOPERS

Even though Mai Li's doctor had called the danazol treatment for her endometriosis "the last card up his sleeve," and they thought waiting six months before trying to conceive again would be devastating, it turned out to be a much-needed vacation.

MAI LI: The vacation for me was a vacation from the pressure of conceiving, a vacation from temperature charts, a vacation from hoping my period wouldn't come—with danazol you don't get a period. It was a vacation from scheduled sex and, more importantly, the pressure to have sex work.

ROY: That was kind of a nice time-out, but it was going to end in six months and we would be back on the road again of pursuing pregnancy. I felt this was a time we can't conceive, so let's do other things. So we rented a house in the country for weekends and the summer, and we started a business together.

MAI LI: Roy is not just my husband, he's my buddy, my best friend. We are very much a team—I feel very connected to him.

ROY: We even had a team spirit about sex. After we had sex, I would literally get down on my hands and knees a few inches from Mai Li's crotch and yell, "Go, sperm, go!" I know it sounds weird, but under the circumstances, it was a way of relieving anxiety and coping.

We followed the book on sex, we did everything we were supposed to do. We were often tired and exhausted, but we made love on the nights we were supposed to.

MAI LI: There were times I wasn't in the mood or was too tired. However, I'm very ambitious and very driven, so even if I was not in the mood or tired I never accepted it as an excuse not to do it.

Since every other night wasn't working, I decided it had to be every night preovulation. At Roy's fortieth birthday party I showed my temperature chart, which had been very erratic, to a doctor friend who also had a fertility problem. She looked at it and said, "Not bad for a man of forty!"

ROY: There were a few times I had problems, but basically we had a good sex life.

MAI LI: The problems we did have were more related to emotions than to sex. When we were at different ends of the emotional spectrum, hope–despair, that was when the conflicts became most acute. When I was feeling hopeful and he felt like throwing in the towel, he got crazy and said things to me like, "What are we doing this for if there's no hope?"

ROY: For the most part, however, I was optimistic. But it was difficult to maintain that optimism in the face of repeated defeat. That whole period was probably the most painful period of my life. But there was no question that we were in this together. We got married to have a family together, and this was just a stumbling block on that road. There were moments of humor, moments of sadness and pain, there was pathos, there was love—the full gamut of feelings. Fortunately, the commitment to each other was stronger than the negative components.

MAI LI: The good that came out of this horrible experience was that our marriage was tested in ways I don't think other relationships ever are, and we had the opportunity to be supportive to each other and work through something together and to really experience a lot of emotions together. I think our marriage came out stronger because of this.

LONG-TERM EFFECTS ON THE MARRIAGE

Most couples with fertility problems find that their marriages survive surprisingly well. Many, in fact, believe their relationships are stronger as a result of having survived this crisis together.

But not all couples agree that infertility strengthens their relationship. In fact, the mere suggestion that that might be the case angers some people.

> There is this notion that whatever doesn't kill me makes me stronger—and almost becomes a good thing. People like to see things in a positive light, and a lot of people say, "Oh, it's bringing us closer together"—they may be just trying to gloss over the trouble and ignore the reality of how divisive and painful infertility can be. It may be that those people had a different experience than we did. We didn't handle it well, or I didn't handle it well, and it ended up being a problem that made us fight and pushed us apart. It seems clear to me that there's more harm than good done. I mean, who needs it? Essentially, I don't think bad things are good for you—I think bad things are bad for you.

But even this man conceded that in the long run, when they were able to confront their problem together, things did work out.

> It didn't pull us together, partly because there was nothing to do together until we decided to try to adopt, and then we began to pull together and work on it together. That was a

positive thing—it was a tremendous relief, and it was exciting and it was a project, it was something we could do.

There are, unfortunately, some marriages that don't survive infertility. But they may have fallen apart even without a fertility problem. All couples have problems—it is their skill in dealing with those problems that largely determines whether their marriages survive. One woman wound up getting separated after fourteen years of marriage.

The effect of infertility on our marriage wasn't very good, let me tell you. I mean, aside from normal everyday problems, it got worse over the infertility issues because it brought out a lot of other things. Like I accused him of not really supporting the whole infertility thing. He would say, "Look, if you want to do it, fine, but I don't want the responsibility." I can't attribute the failure of our marriage entirely to it, but I think it was a contributing factor because it opened a Pandora's box. But I almost stayed in the marriage because I was very desperate to have a child and it seemed to me like the only way I could do it. I thought, "I'm caught here, so I'll stay longer because I really want to have this child."

Other couples find that their relationships do initially deteriorate, but somehow they are able to pull things together.

Our relationship has gone through cycles—it started off sort of on an even keel and then got dramatically worse. I must confess that when I felt that I was fine and that it was his problem, I felt resentful toward him—that if I married someone else, I would have three children. But then as things progressed and it became apparent that I had a problem, it turns out that he's a better person than I am because he doesn't have these resentful feelings. And in the last eight months, our relationship has become better, better than it ever was. There's a closeness, probably from suffering together and surmounting it.

It's important to remember that although infertility is a difficult period in your life, it's just a temporary situation. Any couple who wants to have a child can do so—if not through their own pregnancy, then through someone else's. And no matter what the outcome of your infertility, you still have your relationship with each other.

> There were times that were very, very hard, and I cried a lot. But it really didn't affect our relationship; it just made for some tense times. And then we would always remember why we were together, who we were, what we wanted in life, and how much we loved each other.

CHAPTER 4

My least favorite holiday of the year is Mother's Day. I hate that holiday. And I never used to.

FAMILY, FRIENDS, AND THE FERTILE WORLD

THE SPANELLIS

Anthony and Sue are both very discreet about their personal lives. At first they didn't mention to their friends that they were trying to get pregnant, much less that they were having difficulty doing so. The first people they spoke to about their infertility were their friends Judy and Rick, who were also having fertility problems. They told them that Anthony had had a varicocelectomy and that he now had a good sperm count, but that they were dismayed because Sue still wasn't pregnant despite the fact she had no diagnosed problem. Judy and Rick suggested that Anthony and Sue join RESOLVE because they would be able to get valuable medical information as well as emotional support.

SUE: Talking to Judy and Rick was the beginning of our opening up to people about our problem. They told us about

61

RESOLVE. It was the first time we heard that there was a support group for infertile couples. We were interested, but still didn't feel we could talk to strangers about this kind of thing.

ANTHONY: We were feeling very isolated. When we talked to Judy and Rick, we felt less isolated. I tend to be someone who doesn't like to talk about any kind of problem, period. There was a certain element of denial. Talking to them did help me open up, because they, having the same problem, knew what we were going through.

SUE: After we had been trying to get pregnant for about a year, I decided to tell my younger sister that we were having trouble conceiving. She and I have always been very close, and she worked for a group of gynecologists, so I thought she would have some understanding of what we were dealing with medically. I mentioned it to my mother about six months later on a visit back home. We were both babysitting for my sister's little boy—it seemed like an appropriate time to mention it. My mother had a lot of trouble with miscarriages, so my parents are very sensitive about such things. My mother is not very open emotionally, but she was very encouraging. I was careful not to give too many details; I didn't tell them that Anthony had the only diagnosed problem because I didn't want them to think badly of him.

I finally told my other sister a few months after that when she was pregnant. I resented her because she was pregnant and she resented me because she had to deal with whether she should work after her child was born and all kinds of issues I wasn't having to deal with. She *demanded* to know why I wasn't trying to get pregnant, and finally I said, "I am trying to get pregnant, but we're having problems." She didn't have too much to say after that.

ANTHONY: My family didn't know a thing. Nobody even knew that I was in the hospital for four days when I had my varicocelectomy. We had an elaborate system that if I got a phone call from my mother, Sue would call me at the hospital and I'd phone my mother from there. I didn't feel comfortable telling my mother; having to deal with my mother was too much—she would have been too upset. I didn't want to talk about it with anybody except Sue.

My sister did ask me once if we were going to have kids. I said, "Yeah, we plan to one day." But I really felt like saying, "I really don't want to tell you nothin'." I have never been comfortable speaking to my family about things like that.

SUE: Obviously—since it took him four years to do it! The problem with Anthony's family was that his sister and brother-in-law complained a lot about their children and told us many times how lucky we were not to have children. That was very difficult for us to hear, so I thought it might be helpful to talk to them about our problem. Also, we had pretty much decided to move ahead on adoption, and we really felt like it wouldn't be quite fair to call them up one day and say "We just adopted a baby!"

ANTHONY: So I called up my mother and told her on the phone that I had something I wanted to talk to her about. And my mother, being Italian, being the person that she is, panicked, thinking it must be something really disastrous, like I have cancer. My brother-in-law immediately called me back to find out what was going on, so I spilled the whole story. I told him we wanted to talk to her about some problems we were having getting pregnant and that we were planning to adopt. My sister also got on the phone—they both were very understanding and supportive. I told my mother the next day at lunch, and she, too, was very supportive.

SUE: Anthony's family had decided by then that we just didn't want to have children, so I think in one sense it was a big relief to them that we wanted to have children. And whether we would be having our own biological child or adopting, either way it was a lot more than they expected. They had assumed, as I had feared, that I was a career woman and not interested in having children. But I felt like it needed to be Anthony's choice as to whether we would say anything.

ANTHONY: I had been afraid to tell them partly because they have never been very supportive of anything that I have ever done in the past. I was afraid they'd blame me for it—that I would be seen as defective. So I was amazed by their reaction—amazed that they were so supportive.

TELLING RELATIVES

Deciding when or what to tell one's family about a fertility problem is a delicate issue. Many people feel the way Anthony did, and would rather not discuss such an intimate matter and sensitive issue with their family; they may want to avoid family interference or may be afraid of a family member's reaction.

I haven't told my mother yet. I guess I'm waiting until it's absolutely definitive that I cannot have my own children, and then I will discuss that with her. I just feel that she's a very fragile kind of guilt-ridden woman and very unaware of her feelings. And her health is going downhill, so I don't want to introduce an additional stress for her to ruminate about. And I don't want to deal with her reaction until I'm sure I have to —I think she will ultimately feel that she is to blame.

Some choose to tell certain family members but not others. One woman explained to me that she had told all the women in her family but hadn't told either of the fathers, because she "assumed that the women can handle it better than the men."

This woman's assumption about the men in her family is, unfortunately, probably correct. However, if men are always shielded from emotionally charged subjects such as infertility, they will continue to have difficulty discussing or understanding such issues.

A couple of years ago I first tried to tell my father we were having fertility problems, but he didn't relate to it. Then after my miscarriage I went to see him and talked to him about it, but again I don't think he understood. I really don't think he got the message until very recently when I told him about the fertility drugs I was taking. And then he said to me, "You don't have to do it for me—I have grandchildren." I said, "Daddy, I'm not doing it for you. Believe me, I'm not doing it for you."

The topic of infertility often makes men feel so uncomfortable or threatened that they make light of the issue or cover up their embarrassment by saying something offensive.

We were all at the dinner table one night and my father was

kind of joking with my husband and said something like, "Let me give you some tips on how to knock her up!" And I told my husband that if he ever had a discussion like that in front of me again, I would divorce him. I was not to be discussed as some kind of breeding cow!

But it's not only the men who say insensitive things to people with fertility problems.

My mother-in-law told me that while she was doing some research, she came upon a very interesting fact—that Napoleon was very much in love with Josephine and the only reason he left her was because she could not have children.

However, most people do find that their families are quite supportive when they do finally confide that they are having fertility problems. The best reaction from family members seems to be one of nonintrusion.

My mother has been very helpful. Probably by not even saying anything, just by listening, giving me a hug, never offering me advice on what we should or shouldn't do, and never saying, "I don't think you should go for any more tests—they make you upset." But just by being there.

My mother is the kind of person who really believes that it's very important to give people their privacy, and I appreciate that. When I said to her, "I'm not getting pregnant. I've been to different specialists. I'm unhappy and I don't know what's going to happen," she didn't get emotionally involved. At first I wondered why she didn't care more. Then I realized that it probably would have been harder on me if she had said, "Oh, you must feel terrible," and on and on. What she said was just, "Oh, I'm glad that you're going to the best doctors, and it sounds like you're doing what you can do." Just sort of supportive and low key. And she never asks me anything. I volunteer information to her, like an update.

STRAINED RELATIONS

Even the best of family relations can become strained when there is a fertility problem, especially when a fertile sibling is involved.

I think I've lost a little of the kind of relationship I used to have with my mother and sister. It will take us a while to get that comfortable again. I think it's been difficult for my sister to go ahead and have children knowing that in doing so it's got to be difficult for me. I have left after many an afternoon with my sister and her children and pulled off to the side of the road and had a good sniffle.

I think this has brought out the sibling rivalry with my sister more than ever. I think she always felt somehow or other inferior to me up 'til now. I'm older than she is and probably more successful than she is, and finally she has something over me—she had a baby.

Most people with fertility problems are usually supersensitive to anything relating to their infertility or someone else's fertility.

I don't feel that my mother has treated me properly. I used to spend a lot of time with my parents—we used to go there practically every Sunday. But now my parents spend Sundays with my sister and her baby. My sister and the baby are always there. My mother would rather spend her days with her wonderful grandchild than listen to her daughter feel miserable about herself.

A seemingly innocent remark or incident can be very upsetting or hurtful. It may provoke a response that seems bizarre to an outsider but is perfectly understandable to anyone who has ever experienced a fertility problem.

On the way home from my fertility doctor, I stopped off at my parents' house. No one was home, but I had a key so I let myself in. I hadn't been home in a while and was taken aback when I saw that the walls were covered with eight-by-ten glossy, colored photos of my sister's new baby, Katie. And on a table was a Mother's Day card that said "To Grandma"—the card was from Katie, a six-month-old baby! I got very upset and shredded it to pieces and then hid the pieces so no one would know what I did.

When I got back to my house, I called my mother and said, "I can't stand coming to your house because it's full of all those pictures of Katie. What about me and my feelings?" My mother said that my sister's pregnancy and baby were not the cause of my infertility. I said, "But you have no space for pictures of my baby if I ever have one. I want you to put up an empty picture frame on the living room wall representing my longed-for child." She said she would think about it and then told my father. He said, "No way!" and told me I was crazy.

THE FELDMANS

Lisa and Eric decided that they would mention their infertility to only a few people. But they also decided not to give full details to anybody; they would say that they both had a fertility problem and were both seeing fertility specialists. No one was to be told how serious it was—that Eric's problem was probably untreatable.

LISA: All our relatives knew that the reason we got married was to have children. The first twenty toasts at our wedding were to the bris [circumcision ceremony]! So when I wasn't pregnant after a few months, most people assumed that something must be wrong, but we never said anything at that point. After a while, my older sister who had had a fertility problem for eighteen years started offering me advice that I didn't want to hear. She started pushing me to go to doctors because I denied that we were seeing specialists. I didn't think it was any of her business.

And then my mother started putting pressure on me. The thing that pissed me off was that one day when I went to visit her, she showed me a baby quilt she had started making. That got me really upset and angry, so I said to her, "Mom, you're putting pressure on me." I told her she should stop because we were trying to get pregnant, we were seeing specialists, and she would be the first to know if and when we had good news. She was very sympathetic, but said she would continue making the quilt—she said it would take her a long time to finish!

ERIC: I had to tell my mother something when the urologist asked me what diseases I had had as a child. I told her the bare minimum—that it was something we had to know for our fertility doctor. She was afraid to ask any questions; she waited until we gave her information. She was waiting for her grandchild, but never put direct pressure on us.

LISA: My teenaged niece and nephew are the only ones who keep asking us when we're going to have children—we never said anything to them about our problem. One day, at a family get-together, we were playing a game called "Scruples" with my niece and nephew. My nephew picked a card with a question for me to answer. He read the card to me—it said, "You want to have a child of your own but you find out your mate is infertile. Do you divorce him?"

ERIC: Lisa said jokingly, "Of course!" I felt my blood pressure shooting way up and I turned beet red. We avoided looking at each other because we knew we would crack up laughing—or crying.

The only friends I told about my infertility were my partner, who is also a good friend, and my best man. I told them everthing except that the infertility was absolute.

LISA: I felt he was lucky to have those two friends to speak to; I didn't have anybody. I told my friends that we were going to a fertility doctor, but they all assumed it was me. I really wanted to talk to somebody about what we were going through, but I couldn't because it was a secret. I didn't feel it was my place to talk about Eric's medical problem. The only way I could talk to people was if I lied, so it was easier to just shut up.

We went out to dinner one night with Eric's sister, who is a lesbian, and her lover. I had gotten to the point where I was desperate to talk to somebody about what we were going through. Eric and I are very close to them both, and they are both psychotherapists, so I decided that we should tell them the truth. But Eric said no to that idea.

ERIC: I didn't understand Lisa's need to talk about the problem. After all, I was the one with the medical problem. During dinner, the conversation turned to babies. My sister and her lover told us that they were also trying to get pregnant—by artificial insemination! So we wound up telling them that I had a serious fertility problem. I realized the need to say, "I can't go through this thing by myself." It turned out to be a relief—it was just what I needed.

LISA: It was good for both of us to have someone we loved to confide in. It made us feel less isolated. They were both loving and supportive, and since they were not having any luck with their artificial inseminations, they were also able to identify with our frustration.

ERIC: Once I started talking to them I just couldn't stop talking about it—it was like letting go of this enormous secret I had had for so long. It was such a relief. The response I got from my sister was the response I wanted from my partner and friends. I wanted to be hugged and held and to have somebody say, "It'll be OK, this is not what you're about." And my sister was able to do that. But I needed that from my men friends—I really needed men. Unfortunately I always get let down by men. Men often act like shmucks, and I have a lot of trouble dealing with them when it gets down to feelings. Men come with a lot of baggage. And I've been surrounded by women all my life. My shrink is even a woman. It's funny, but through this whole thing I've dreamed about my dad a lot—I've needed a man to talk to.

TELLING FRIENDS

Unfortunately, many people with fertility problems are disappointed with their friends' reactions to their problems. The major reason for this seems to be that unless someone has experienced a fertility problem, they cannot truly understand the emotional upheaval it causes. The reactions of friends often fall into two categories, pity and insensitivity—neither of which is helpful for the infertile person.

I was having lunch with two old friends from high school, both of whom had children. They said, "Well, have you given any thought to having children?" And I said, "Yes, I have." And they said, "Well, what's the problem?" And I said, "Have you ever heard the word infertility?" And they tried to find out what it was all about. It was all very embarrassing and uncomfortable. They were feeling sorry for me, and I can't stand being pitied—so I wound up feeling defensive.

When I told my friends, many would say, "Oh, you're crazy, it's no big deal. I don't know what the hell you're trying to get pregnant for—kids are awful." Those are the ones who have at least two. Other people give me the old "relax" trip. In the beginning I used to get real angry and not say anything. Now I just lash out. I've been very verbal in telling people off, especially people who said to me after we adopted our baby, "Well, now you'll get pregnant."

You may find that the easiest way to deal with sensitive questions or insensitive remarks is to have ready answers or retorts.

At first when people asked me if I was going to have children I used to say, "We're trying." Later I just said, "I'm infertile." And then I got to the point where I would say, "I'm barren." I did it on purpose, because when you say that you're trying, they ask you four thousand questions, but when you come out and say, "I'm sterile" or "I'm barren," they just shut up!

This adds an element of control to a situation where you probably feel out of control. In addition, this type of straightforward response may help people become more sensitive to the problem of infertility and be more careful about what they say to you and others in the future.

If you are going to be in a social situation where you know you are likely to be greeted by unwelcome or unanswerable questions, insensitive comments, or unsolicited advice, it is better to prepare for them ahead of time. You can even try roleplaying with your spouse. Or you can make a game of trying to guess who will ask what insensitive question or make what absurd remark—you might find it fun as well as helpful. If you realize ahead of time that Aunt Edna is probably going to ask when the two of you are ever going to stop being selfish and have a baby so your mother can finally become a grandmother, and Uncle Harry will tell you to relax and take a vacation, and Cousins Mimi and Pam are going to tell you that if you adopt you'll get pregnant, and your college roommate will tell you you're better off not having kids because they're nothing but trouble, and your mother-in-law will tell you that you're lucky you miscarried because the baby was probably deformed to begin with—instead of being upset when it happens, you can say to yourself or your spouse, "I knew she would say that," and have your response ready.

If someone gives you unsolicited or insensitive advice, you might try saying that infertility is a personal matter and you are under the care of a very competent physician. They probably won't bother you again. Infertility counselor Roselle Shubin suggests if someone asks you when you are going to have children, you can just say, "We're having some problems and we're getting medical help, and you can also help by not asking us questions about it for now because it's a painful area for us to discuss." A statement of fact like that should end the discussion without hurting anyone's feelings.

Another common problem with friends who don't have fertility problems is that they cannot understand the constant preoccupation and obsession with infertility—they get bored or threatened or both.

We went away to a country inn with another couple we were very close to. At dinner we started discussing our fertility problems, and my friend said, "You should just forget about it for a while; you're putting too much emphasis on it—you talk about it all the time!" And my husband said, "I guess if you're not going through this you don't know how painful it is. It's the most important thing to us right now." I was very hurt and angry—that here was a good friend who would not tolerate this painful period in my life. Our friendship started to wane after that, and now we don't have a friendship any more.

According to RESOLVE's president, Beverly Freeman, "One of the heartrending aspects of infertility is that people can find out who their real friends are." Although it's difficult for someone who has never been through infertility to understand fully, they can still listen and be supportive. Ms. Freeman says that one of the advantages of organizations such as RESOLVE is that you can meet new people and make new friends with other couples who are just as sensitive to and preoccupied with infertility as you are. And they will definitely not be of the "just relax" school!

THE COOPERS

After Mai Li was on danazol to treat her endometriosis for six months, she was able to start trying to conceive again. Even though those six months were a kind of vacation from the pressure of conceiving, both Roy and Mai Li were happy to start trying again. But they also felt tremendous pressure because if danazol works, usually it's within the six months following treatment. Their doctor told them that if she didn't conceive during those six months, he would want to do another laparoscopy. Those months were a very trying time for them both.

MAI LI: I was beginning to feel less optimistic. The prognosis was not very good; endometriosis was a real obstacle to overcome. Also, surgery was such a bad experience that a lot of rage and self-pity started coming out because I had to go through this ordeal when other people didn't And there was no guarantee I would get pregnant after all I had been through. I mostly felt rage, sadness, and panic.

ROY: Prior to having this problem with infertility, I would have been Joe Schmo out there who would have said, "What's all this fuss about having your own kid? Why don't you just adopt?" I never would have imagined that with all the problems in the world, this would be so painful. So I could understand the outside world's inability to see and understand the pain.

MAI LI: There was a part of Roy that still had his foot in the fertile world. I lost that footing! I felt the fertile world was callous, cruel, stupid.

Everybody in Roy's family knew that we were infertile and struggling with this problem, and that I had had surgery and everything. Around the time we were trying to decide if I should have another laparoscopy, we went to a family party, and Roy's Aunt Edna was there. Her husband had died a few months before, and we hadn't seen her since the funeral. Aunt Edna came up to me at the party and said, "How are you doing?" I said, "Basically fine, but we're still going through a lot of problems trying to conceive, and I may have to have more surgery." She said, "Oh, that's too bad. I hope it works out," and then she said, "Would you like to see pictures of my new grandchild? I'm so happy I have a grandchild." I quickly changed the subject, but I was furious. I felt like saying to her, "Would you like to see pictures of my husband? I'm so happy I have a husband who is not dead!" But nobody would say to someone who just lost a husband, "I'm so happy my husband is alive!" So they shouldn't turn to an infertile person and say, "I'm so happy I just had a grandchild." Why grind your foot into another person's misery? But they don't see it that way.

A few minutes later, my mother-in-law came up to me and said, "Did you see pictures of Aunt Edna's grandchild?" And I said, "No." And she said, "Should I get them for you?" And I said, "I don't want to look at pictures of babies." And she said, "Oh, my God, I'm so sorry!" Later she came over to me during the party and said, "I feel terrible—I feel so stupid."

ROY: I was proud of Mai Li for speaking out like that. In the beginning I was not always supportive or understanding of Mai Li's difficulty with pregnant women and babies. One weekend a friend of mine, Mark, and his pregnant wife, June, were coming in from the East Coast and wanted to visit us. I wanted them to come over to dinner, but Mai Li refused to see them. I couldn't understand not seeing them just because of her pregnancy. We're very close emotionally, and I didn't want the infertility to interfere with our relationship.

MAI LI: We had a terrible fight. I had no interest in seeing a pregnant woman, friend or no friend. I didn't want to have someone else's success flaunted in my face. I felt Roy should see them on his own, since the pregnancy didn't seem to bother him.

ROY: They are very sensitive people; Mark even called up ahead of time and asked if it would upset Mai Li to see June pregnant.

MAI LI: I was furious that he asked Roy if I would mind being around June. Of course I would mind, but for him to verbalize my sensitivity made me furious—it made me feel like an invalid to be pitied. But I was also touched by Mark's sensitivity about the issue. His asking Roy if I would be upset gave my sensitivity to pregnant women some credence, some validity. I used that question to confirm to Roy that I wasn't so crazy to feel that way, because even Mark and June could understand how I might feel about pregnant women—even someone in the fertile world agreed that I was normal. For Roy to pressure me into seeing them was wrong. I was really angry at him.

ROY: I felt Mai Li was entitled to her feelings, but that they shouldn't affect our relationships with friends; these were friends of mine who came all the way from Boston to see us. Here was a couple she could gain strength from being around because they were sympathetic—they were a couple we could openly discuss things with.

MAI LI: I finally gave in because I felt guilty—Mark is Roy's oldest and dearest friend. I pouted a lot before they came over. I had some emotional pain, but the evening was tolerable. I rose to the occasion and put on an Academy Award-winning performance.

ROY: In retrospect, I realize I made light of Mai Li's pain. I shouldn't have forced her into something she felt so strongly about. I just didn't want infertility to affect our lives to the point where we couldn't see certain people.

MAI LI: There was no objective reason why Roy shouldn't have had dinner alone with them, spend days with them, and for me not to be involved. Where Roy's and my close relationship usually worked in our favor, it also worked against us in cases like this where we were expected to socialize as a unit. Here is an instance where our closeness caused us grief.

A pregnancy was devastating to me—it destroyed me—and I was angry about Roy's lack of understanding about that. I didn't want anything to do with pregnant women. I had fantasies of them having miscarriages, or stillborn or deformed babies. I wanted their pregnancies to fail so that they would be failures just like I was.

ROY: As time went on, I was able to identify more with Mai Li's feelings. I wanted to punch pregnant women right in their big fat bellies. I also wanted pregnant couples to fail—I wanted them to understand the degree of pain that we were going through. But I also felt happy when someone who had really struggled with infertility became pregnant. They were more deserving.

MAI LI: If I felt a person was undeserving, that bothered me the most. If I was competitive with a person on any level and they became pregnant, that also bothered me.

My friend Amy and I had talked about getting pregnant about the same time, but I started trying a year before she did. By then I was clearly infertile and going through a lot of crap. She said, "I'm going to try and get pregnant next month because I want to have a baby in the spring," and the next month she was pregnant! I tried to suppress a lot of my hostility. I even went to see the baby in the hospital. Then I went to a dinner party at her home and, of course, she showed off the baby. I was overcome with grief and envy. I felt like sobbing, but I held back my tears. A few weeks later we had lunch together and Amy said, "Why don't you and Roy come for dinner next Saturday night?" I said, "We're busy." And she said, "Tell me what Saturday night you're not busy." And I said, "Look, I don't think I can come to your house." She asked why not and I said, "Because, as you know, I've been struggling to become pregnant for two years and it's painful for me to visit people with babies." As I was telling her this, I started to cry. She was shocked and got very flustered and embarrassed and turned bright red and said, "Oh, my God, I had no idea!" She is a very bright and sensitive person and was embarrassed that she hadn't realized how much pain she had inadvertently caused me. After that, we occasionally spoke on the phone, but she never talked about my coming over again.

DEALING WITH THE FERTILE WORLD

Perhaps the least understood but most emotionally charged issue for the infertile couple is how to deal with pregnant women and newborn babies. Common reactions to seeing a pregnant woman are often a combination of envy, hate, hostility, and wonder. Infertile women, more than men, become acutely aware of pregnant women. As one woman told me, "It seems like I have tunnel vision for pregnant women; they just seem to be popping up everywhere."

When someone is infertile, they often think the whole world is pregnant except for them. Even unmarried teenagers and undernourished women in India manage to get pregnant with no problems. Why can't *they?* Why should something so easy for most people to accomplish be so difficult for them? It is not difficult to understand why someone with a fertility problem has a hard time dealing with pregnant women.

If I'm on a bus and a pregnant woman comes in I will never give her my seat—that's how I get out my hostility. Somebody could be delivering on the bus, and I won't give her my seat.

Very often these hostile feelings lead to fantasies of violence against the pregnant woman.

When I see pregnant women, I want to kill—take out a knife and stab every pregnant woman. You wonder what about her makes her capable of having children—what does she have that I don't have?

These violent fantasies, while they may seem extreme and incomprehensible to the fertile world, can help you vent your anger and hostility in a harmless manner. Even when the hostile feelings get acted out, they are usually quite innocuous.

I work right across the street from a maternity shop, and sometimes I want to kick the window or stone it or something, but of course I never do. But sometimes when pregnant women come out of there looking for a cab, I jump into the first one. Even if they look like they are due tomorrow, I have absolutely no guilt about taking that cab.

A pregnant woman may be considered particularly undeserving because everything seems to come too easily for her in life.

I was very ticked off when Princess Di got pregnant. That really bothered me. It even bothered me more than my friend being pregnant at the same time. I remember the day I heard about Princess Di. I was a nut. I couldn't believe it. My God, she gets knocked up the second month she's married! How dare she!

Some feel ambivalent about pregnant women rather than purely hostile.

I feel very mixed, very ambivalent around pregnant women. I mean, I live vicariously through their pregnancies. But I'm also envious. I wish it were me. I have such a yearning. I'm past the point of hating them—it's gone so far beyond that because I've been so angry about it; I think I've worked that through. When I see them the first thing I see is not the face, but this big stomach. And I just say to myself, "Oh, I can't wait until that's me. I wish that was me. Maybe one day it will happen."

And there are some women who, when they see a pregnant woman, experience a sense of wonder or awe.

When I see pregnant women, I want to run up to them and ask how they did it—"By the way, what day did you have sex on to produce this? Was it the fourteenth or the sixteenth? Do you have a twenty-eight-day cycle or a thirty-two-day cycle? Did you do it in the morning? Did you lie in bed afterwards? Did you eat five million oysters?" I mean, it's this incredible thing that's beyond my grasp, and I want to find out.

Pregnant Friends and Relatives

Anonymous pregnancies are one thing, but when a friend or relative becomes pregnant, that's another story. As one woman told me, "Pregnant women in the street have no relation to my life. But the one thing that disconcerts me is when a close friend gets pregnant." Others feel that the pregnancy of a relative is the hardest to take because it is "too close for comfort," as another woman put it. It's often very hard to deal with a relative's pregnancy because there may be a long history of rivalry between the siblings or cousins.

It doesn't matter whether the pregnant woman is a friend or relative; there is no easy way to be told about the pregnancy of someone close to you.

I have a cousin in Canada who is five years older than I am—she's my role model. She's a lawyer and happily married. She has two children who are beautiful, smart, cute, and everything. I love her and admire her a great deal. She knows about our fertility problem. I got a call from her one night around eleven-thirty, and we were already asleep. We hardly ever talk on the phone. I was totally caught off guard. She said, "Hi—I just wanted to let you know before you heard it from your mom, I'm pregnant." I said, "Oh, congratulations. You must be really excited. That's really wonderful. I didn't know you wanted another kid." I was totally appropriate, but it was really hard on me. I had sweat dripping down my arms. And then later I realized how angry I was at her. She didn't have to phone me up at night. She could have written me a letter. It would have been much better to read it, so I didn't have to respond to her right away. Because what am I going to say to her? "You bitch! Don't you have enough already?" I have to be appropriate. I love her. I don't wish bad things for her.

The pregnancy of either a friend or a relative cannot be ignored. Some action has to be taken, even if it's inaction, because the relationship may be at stake.

When friends of mine are pregnant, I can't stand it, but I feel like I have to do something to preserve some modicum of friendship—but I just can't stand it.

Unfortunately, whatever you choose to do about a pregnant friend or relative, it is likely to cause some pain—either to yourself if you spend time with her, or to the pregnant person if you choose to ignore her. If you choose the former and see her, you may temporarily be jeopardizing your emotional stability. If you choose the latter and ignore her, you may be jeopardizing your friendship—the choices certainly aren't great! So how do you resolve the conflict?

Socializing in the Fertile World

Some choose to grin and bear it when visiting pregnant women or new mothers. But, as one woman put it, "It's very difficult to be happy for and take an interest in somebody you're basically jealous of." Infertility counselor Roselle Shubin suggests, "Ask yourself what kinds of socializing you can handle and enjoy and what might cause you too much distress. You should then be very selective in accepting invitations."

This same advice holds especially when it comes to showers, birthday parties, christenings, or any other social occasion that is likely to cause you pain because of the presence of babies, small children, pregnant women, or prying relatives. Remember, your absence from one of these occasions may cause your hostess or the guest of honor a few seconds of distress, but they will be so preoccupied with the party and the rest of the guests that they are likely not to give you much more than a fleeting thought. You, on the other hand, will be some place you don't want to be, and may suffer for it for hours.

You should ask yourself if it's really worth hours of your own unhappiness just to save someone else a few moments of disappointment over your absence. And if you choose to explain why you are not going, if the person's feelings are hurt, then they clearly do not understand or respect your feelings. And finally, you should ask yourself what you are going to accomplish by going.

I did make the mistake of going to my niece's first birthday party after my second miscarriage. I felt, well, it's my sister. But when I stepped in the house I knew I had made the wrong decision. I was crying inside and just holding myself together. That's all I could do. And I never experienced that before—but I have since.

It was very dumb of my sister not to think it through; I think I would have. She had lots of mothers there with babies. And an old friend was there seven months pregnant. No one ever told me. At first I wasn't sure—she's overweight. It took me a few minutes to stare at her—my mouth must have been open—to realize that she was pregnant. It hit me that no one knew what to say, because if they called me up and said, "Sherry's pregnant"—you think, how terrible that is. Why do they have to do that? And if they don't tell you—I mean, I understood, but it was like a knife in my heart. I was just shaking, but I refused to make a scene.

At that point I decided I would never go through that again. It's my life, and it's too painful. I feel right now that I come first. I will not subject myself to people who are pregnant or have young children. If they don't understand, it's their problem, because I don't care right now. But that will pass. And if those friendships don't last, I don't care.

Protecting yourself from pain is not selfish, it's sensible. It's also important to remember that you will not feel this way forever. Once your infertility is resolved, you will find it easier to go to social events where there are babies or pregnant women present. You will no longer feel the same anger or anguish you most likely now feel in their company.

In the meantime, you might be pleasantly surprised to find out that there are people out there in the fertile world who do understand your pain and agree that you shouldn't have to suffer unnecessarily.

I could not bring myself to hand-make a shower present for my sister's second child—something I could do with great enthusiasm for the first one. And I tried and tried and I decided that it was a matter of discipline; I was just being silly and emotional. Finally my mother said to me, "This is unnecessary. And it doesn't mean beans to your sister. Why are you doing this to yourself?"

And as careful as you may be to avoid painful situations, you can't protect yourself against all the hurts imposed by the fertile world.

I miscarried in the fourth month of my pregnancy. And five months later, the month my baby was supposed to be born, I started getting *American Baby Magazine.* I wrote to everybody and couldn't get the magazine stopped. Getting the first issue was especially horrendous. Also, because I was on their mailing list, I got free coupons in the mail for diapers, formula, baby powder, you name it. Now I'm writing them and telling them they had better send me the magazines and coupons because I've adopted a baby!

CHAPTER 5

My mind was not on my career. It was just on holding myself together and getting pregnant. My main goal now is to get pregnant, and that's the most important thing—to see that through. It's become my job.

INFERTILITY
9-TO-5

THE COOPERS

Roy's career as a cinematographer was going well. Except for the episode of not being able to go into a hot tub to do filming—because the heat might affect his sperm count—infertility had little impact on his career. According to Roy, "Work was my salvation. When I was working, it really did take my mind off infertility. I was not consumed with it." Mai Li's story, however, was different. When they first started trying to conceive, Mai Li was an assistant sportswear buyer for a department store in San Francisco, but she didn't like her job and decided to find a better one. She got a new job as head buyer at an exclusive boutique at the same time she was starting her infertility workup.

MAI LI: It was soon after I started my new job that my doctor, Dr. S., recommended surgery because the hysterosalpingogram showed that I had blocked tubes. Dr. S. then informed me that this would not be a routine laparoscopy because more extensive surgery would be needed to remove the adhesions; I would have to be out of work for six weeks. That was very stressful for me, because I had to inform my new boss. So I went to her and said, "Listen, I have to talk to you, I have some bad news for us." She got really nervous because she thought I was going to resign just like the previous head buyer. So she was really relieved that I was just going to be out for six weeks. It was very fortunate that she really liked me.

I told her that the surgery was for gynecological problems; I never mentioned infertility. I felt that since the surgery was elective, she would be unsympathetic and think I was unprofessional to go for surgery so soon after starting a new job.

Roy: Mai Li was also concerned that if she said she was going in for surgery to correct a fertility problem, they would realize she was trying to get pregnant, and that might jeopardize her position.

Mai Li: I planned my surgery to coincide with the Christmas holidays because that's a very slow time for buyers and people are away on vacation a lot anyway. Even though the surgery was very extensive because Dr. S. discovered I had severe endometriosis, I recovered in record time and was able to go back to work part time before the six weeks were up.

Roy: Mai Li had a quick physical recovery, but she got more and more depressed because we weren't getting pregnant, and we knew that danazol treatment was the next step if she still wasn't pregnant in six months.

Mai Li: Sometimes I got so depressed that I couldn't work. I was too preoccupied to be able to concentrate, and that started to become a problem. I had rarely let any personal problems interfere with my work; before I had always been able to put my personal life aside and get my work done. This period was the only time in my career that I was having difficulty doing that. I functioned just enough not to get fired.

I really liked my job, and as time went on I started functioning better and better. But then my boss decided to close the shop, and I had to start looking for a new job.

I answered a lot of ads in the trade paper, and one day I got a call from this guy who said he had received my résumé and wanted to talk to me. I said, "Tell me something about the job," and he said it was for a position as head buyer for a chain of maternity boutiques! It struck me as very funny and ironic. I said, "I don't remember answering any ad for a maternity boutique," and he said that they didn't mention that in the ad. So I kind of laughed and said, "You *really* have the wrong person—you don't know how *wrong* I am for this job!" And he said, "Why do you say that?" Then I realized I was being unprofessional, so I told him that I had no experience in buying maternity clothes. He said, "We're looking for someone with no experience in that area because we want a fresh approach."

For about five minutes I tried to talk him out of interviewing me, which I sensed made him want to talk to me more. He finally said, "Listen, it won't hurt for us to meet and talk," so I agreed to an interview. I was feeling psychologically better, because by then we had started to look into adoption. Also, I had just been on a lot of interviews in rat-infested lofts with creeps that laughed at my salary requirements. So I felt I had nothing to lose.

When I went for the interview, everyone was very nice, very professional, very corporate—both the men and women wore suits, and the offices were beautiful, with magnificent views of San Francisco. When I gave them a salary range, they offered me the top of the range! It seemed too good to be true—except for the fact that I would have to see pregnant models and pick out fashions that would flatter what I at times considered disgusting pregnant bodies. I didn't know if I could handle it. I didn't know what to do.

JOB INTERFERENCE

Infertility can interfere with someone's work and career in several ways. Finding the time (not to mention the boss's understanding) to take off from work for doctors' appointments for fertility tests or treatment can be tricky. Too much time away from the office can jeopardize a career. It may be necessary to find a doctor with a flexible schedule or at times even postpone medical treatment for the sake of the job.

> When I had artificial inseminations, it was a problem because I would sometimes have to get up at the crack of dawn to get to the doctor's office early so I could make it to work on time. But he was very nice and would sometimes see me earlier than his normal hours to help me out because I had a meeting at nine A.M. But it was difficult; I was charging up there in the middle of the day sometimes and I was in a new, stressful job. I also decided not to have a laparoscopy because I had just taken this new job.

If the employee *does* succeed in becoming pregnant, a whole new set of work-related problems can arise, as one psychiatrist with both a part-time job and a private practice found out.

> The first time I was pregnant, nobody knew at work. I just took a day off here and there. After I miscarried, I told people, because I was depressed. The second time I had just taken four weeks' vacation, and on the vacation I had discovered I was pregnant and I was spotting. When I came home I went to this doctor who told me to stay in bed. So I stayed. He said I had to stay in bed until two weeks after the bleeding stopped. So I went back to work for one day and then called up and told them what was going on, and I took a leave of absence. Then I called my patients and said, "I'm not feeling well. I'll see you in two weeks." And then in two weeks I had to call them again because I had another miscarriage.

Both men and women have to worry about taking time off from work for doctors' appointments, but it is usually the women who find that infertility interferes with their work psychologically. Many find that they are so obsessed with or depressed about their infertility, they sometimes have difficulty functioning at work.

> I've done very bad work in the last six months. I've barely been functioning. Doing a good job or being committed to it has become unimportant to me. I don't know what's going to

happen. The work has gotten sloppy, and the kind of work I do is creative; it has to come out of me. And when I'm depressed, I'm burnt out and I don't care. I should be going places and speaking and meeting people and making contacts. And I just haven't. I also lost a great deal of time from work, especially after the last miscarriage.

But infertility can also affect a man's performance on the job. As one baseball player put it, "After I discovered I had a fertility problem, my batting average went way down."

Pregnant Women at Work

When the job involves dealing with pregnant women or new mothers, there is no professionally acceptable way to vent one's hostility or resentment. As a result, the problems at work can become even more exaggerated, as a psychotherapist who had repeated miscarriages discovered.

During the two years that I was really depressed, I was marginally functioning and half the time not listening and being fully productive. A lot of my patients talk about wanting to have children, and I have trouble with that. One of them was pregnant at the same time that I would have been if I hadn't miscarried, and that was really difficult. And another patient is an alcoholic. Her baby was born the same time I miscarried the first time, and that was really difficult for me. She is a terrible mother. I have trouble dealing with her—I keep thinking I'd be so much better a mother than she is.

Dealing with pregnant co-workers also creates problems, and unlike pregnant friends or relatives, pregnant co-workers are visible on a daily basis, so they cannot easily be avoided.

When my assistant gave birth it was devastating. Everybody in the office was running up to me and saying, "Isn't it wonderful about Sally? Have you talked to her, have you seen her?" I think that was one of the most difficult periods. I can't say I hate her, because I love her. But at that time I hated her. And she said that she was going to come up to the office with the baby, and I just really did not want to see that baby. And she is someone I've discussed this with. I mean, she knew every-thing I was going through. And we care about each other. But I really hated her for doing it so easily. She had a naming ceremony, and I just wouldn't be caught dead going. I still don't know what I'm going to do when I see that baby—I dread seeing that baby.

It can be extremely demoralizing when a pregnant co-worker does or says something insensitive, especially if it's work-related.

Another doctor, a colleague of mine, is two-and-a-half months pregnant. She had a patient who got treated with radioactive iodine for an overactive thyroid. She called me up and asked me what my pregnancy status was and whether I was willing to see the patient who was sick one week after being treated with the radioactive iodine; since she was pregnant, she didn't want to see the patient. And I really resented that—I mean, I didn't want to be asked whether I was pregnant or whether I wasn't pregnant, whether I was trying this month or whether I wasn't trying this month. There were several other doctors she could have called. I just don't want to be the sterile one in the group that you call up when you don't want to be exposed to radiation!

Working with Children

Another potential problem area is a job that entails working with young children. People with fertility problems may find themselves in a situation where they become emotionally involved or emotionally overcome, as one doctor discovered when she did her residency in pediatrics.

Last week I went to see a young boy on pediatrics. He has spina bifida [a genetic disease that causes permanent crip-pling], so his legs are weak and he has to walk on crutches. He's nine years old and was in the hospital with severe burns on his feet. When I heard about him I thought, God, what a terrible thing to have a child like that—what a burden. And I went to see him, and I walked in and I fell in love. He was beautiful and cute and so bright. I was in love—he was just the cutest little boy. And I looked at his feet and they were terrible. His mother had put him in a burning hot bathtub to punish him because he was incontinent of feces—he has no neurological control, and she fucking burned him! I can't believe it. And I have to struggle like this to have a child! And she's abusing this brilliant, beautiful, wonderful child. I would like to kill her!

Working with children on a professional level, although at times unsettling, can ultimately be a rewarding experience for someone longing to have a child of her own.

You can't condemn kids because they're born and you don't have any children. You just love them for what they are. They understand a lot more about what's going on than you think. Even those questions like, "Do you have kids?" Their reactions are a lot more sensible than some adults.

I think I have an advantage working with children—it does take a certain amount of maternal feelings, even though it's on a professional level. It's enjoyable. I'm in an enviable position. I think it's more enjoyable for me than it would be to be an aunt or visit a friend's child. When I have these kids, they're *my* kids.

THE SPANELLIS

When Anthony and Sue got married, Anthony was working as a computer programmer, but started additional training in order to qualify as a systems analyst. Sue was in charge of a small program in the Bronx for handicapped adults. She was working on her Ph.D. in psychology and hoped to eventually get a job that combined clinical work and research.

SUE: When I was first trying to get pregnant, I was thinking about changing jobs, and for a while I decided that it didn't make sense to try to make a change at that point. There were some advantages to being in the job I was in. I figured I would get pregnant in a few months, and it was a good job to be pregnant in because it wasn't too demanding, and the maternity benefits were excellent.

As time went on and I still wasn't pregnant, I started to think that my trying to get pregnant was not something I

should base my life plans on. But I figured that when I finished my Ph.D. I'd be in a better position to move on to a new
job. I finally got my doctorate two years later, but by then I
was starting a whole new battery of fertility tests with my new
doctor. I was also doing a little college teaching as well as
working full time, and I was tired. I also realized that I was
going to be starting on Pergonal, so it wasn't a good time to
change jobs; I knew I would have to have a lot of doctors'
appointments and blood tests during that time.

ANTHONY: Once I became qualified to be a systems analyst,
I started looking for a new job and got one very quickly, but it
was in Westchester and meant that we both had to commute
to work, but only one of us could use the car. We decided I
should get the car because my new office was less accessible to
public transportation than Sue's office. That caused a bit of a
problem for us, as well as the fact that I was able to change
jobs and Sue wasn't. She felt envious and I felt guilty—I had
the freedom and she didn't.

SUE: I did resent Anthony to some extent—I had worked
so hard all these years going to school to get my doctorate
and then found myself in a position where I couldn't change
jobs or even look for a new job. Anthony, who has only a
bachelor's degree, which is just fine with me, had just qualified as a systems analyst, and he could just go out and get
another better job. I had a Ph.D. and was a qualified psychologist and I couldn't do that! Sometimes I asked him not to talk
so much about his new job. I just didn't need to hear it.

ANTHONY: I realized how hard she had worked to get her
Ph.D., and I was annoyed she didn't get an opportunity to
use it.

SUE: Right before I went on Pergonal, I thought that just
maybe I could still make a job change. I went for a job interview for a research position I was very much interested in.
They told me they were very interested in me and wanted me
for a second interview, but by then I had started Pergonal and
realized I could not start a new job and be in a position to
have to have blood tests three mornings per week at midcycle,
get to work late, and sometimes be even later because I would
need an exam or sonogram or insemination. So it was an

issue of priorities, and what we needed to give priority to was dealing with the issue of whether or not I would ever get pregnant. Anthony was disappointed that I couldn't take the job.

ANTHONY: I felt very angry and upset about how much this damn infertility had taken over our lives and that Sue was still in her old job.

SUE: Anthony changed jobs just when we were starting on Pergonal, and his job meant that I wasn't going to have the car, which made me feel even less in control because I had been using the car to get to work.

ANTHONY: When I started in Manhattan, there was no problem getting away for doctors' appointments. But when I started commuting to Westchester, getting away for appointments was a real pain, even though I had a car.

SUE: The most difficult times were when we were doing the artificial inseminations with Anthony's sperm and I was on Pergonal, and we would have to wait for the hormone blood test results that would indicate whether my estradiol level was high enough for me to ovulate.

ANTHONY: Sue would call me up at work the minute she knew the results of the estradiol tests and say, "We have to do it today." I would have to go up to my boss and say, "I have a doctor's appointment in Manhattan, I need an extended lunch hour." I would then get in the car, drive all the way down to Manhattan, hassle with the traffic, leave a sperm deposit, and drive back up—an hour-and-a-half round trip in good traffic!

SUE: And there were times I had to have a blood test in the morning, take a bus all the way to the Bronx, not get to work until ten-thirty, talk to my doctor at three, and find out that it looked like probably it was a day we should do an insemination, so I would have to turn around and get the bus back to the city and then go back to work. It was really disruptive, and I wanted to stop the inseminations.

Getting away for the blood tests and inseminations became a significant issue at work. I'm in charge of the office and I run the outpatient program, and I'm the kind of person who feels like I can't have certain expectations and standards for my staff and then not follow them myself. So it was very out of character for me to come in to work late several days a week.

I decided I was going to talk to people at work because they knew something was wrong. I also knew I needed to feel less isolated and to give myself more sources of support. Paula, the second person I talked with, said to me, "I think I'd better tell you something I just found out. I'm pregnant." I just sat there, and I really had to work very hard to stay in control. But she was great; we had a lot of good talks. Still, it was hard for me to deal with the fact that she was pregnant, and hard for her to deal with the fact that I was having these problems while she was pregnant.

I ended up feeling even more glad that I had talked to the people at work about my fertility problems, because they were able to be particularly sensitive in dealing with Paula's pregnancy around me.

Telling People at Work

The issue of whether to tell people at work that you are having a fertility problem is difficult. Some, like Sue, find that letting people know they are having problems helps them feel less isolated as well as providing a rationale for some seemingly irrational or uncharacteristic behavior. On the other hand, some women may find that their jobs are jeopardized if their employers realize they are trying to get pregnant.

According to psychotherapist Dr. Kate Gorman, "There isn't any one particular answer—if you tell people at work, it means you're not harboring a painful secret, and you can be more open about what your needs are in terms of time off for doctors' appointments or other things. If you don't tell, you have a place where you don't have to face your infertility all the time—there aren't people asking you how the appointment went, or whether your husband's sperm count is up. Work can be an oasis from infertility."

MAKING CAREER DECISIONS

Infertility has the unfortunate ability to put people's lives on hold. It's difficult under the best of circumstances to make career decisions or changes, but when you add the variable of uncertainty over pregnancy, it becomes even more difficult. The infertile woman has no idea *when* or even *if* she will ever get pregnant or adopt a child—either of which could take her months or years. Under those circumstances, it often seems easier to keep putting off career decisions in the hope that a pregnancy will come to the rescue.

I kept thinking every Christmas, Good, I'll either have a kid by next Christmas or be pregnant, and I won't have to work here any more. Meanwhile, every year I'm back again.

I kept expecting to get pregnant—that's why I kept this job. I keep saying I don't like what I do. I need to go job hunting. I need to get a new job. On the other hand, if I get pregnant, I'm in a wonderful position because I can take time off. I can walk to work—I would be four blocks away from my baby. If I'm going to have children, I'm working at the perfect place. And so I delay doing anything.

Taking a job or staying in a job because of maternity benefits may seem like a good idea at the time, but can be especially frustrating when it is the other women who become pregnant and reap those benefits.

I was really thinking about changing jobs, but there were some advantages to staying in this job—I figured I would get pregnant in a few months and there wouldn't be any problem in taking a leave for several months after the baby was born. That was two-and-a-half years ago . . . One of the most difficult things in dealing with pregnancies at work was that as the person in charge, I had to be very objective over issues like maternity leave, and sometimes I bent over backwards to show myself I was going to be objective even though I had all these subjective hostile feelings.

However, some people, like Sue, realistically have to delay career decisions or changes because infertility treatment makes it virtually impossible for them to make the change.

I haven't been able to work full time ever since the beginning of this fertility problem, because how can you when you're taking off for this and that and the other thing? And going three times a week for AIH, and then this time for a blood test and that time for a postcoital test. I don't know how anyone can work full time and actually do all this and then take time off for a laparoscopy or tubal surgery. So I didn't look for full-time work. And part-time work is working full time for part-time pay!

Many women with fertility problems feel in retrospect that they have made the wrong career decisions.

If I had thought that I would have all these fertility problems, I think I would have done everything much faster. I wouldn't have wasted all those years. I regret going through the master's in urban planning instead of going to law school. I did that because it was the kind of program where I could go part time in case I got pregnant, instead of law school, where you have to go full time.

It's especially frustrating because they lose on two counts—they have neither the career nor the child they hoped for.

I took this job because I felt it would be a perfect job for me to have while I had my family. So I took the job and the job sucks. And I don't have a family. So now I'm angry at myself, because I never should have made a decision based on something I had no control over. If I'd known when I finished my fellowship that I would be unable to have children for the next two or three years, I never would have taken that job. I would have worked on my career.

Some people try to work out their frustrations over infertility by incorporating it into their professional lives, by writing about the subject, or by working with infertile people. This is an excellent solution for some, but others find it extremely difficult to combine work and infertility, as one writer discovered.

Since I was so personally involved with infertility, and a lot of people were interested in the topic, I thought it would be a good idea to do a story on infertility. It turned out to be a terrible experience. It put my professional and personal lives in conflict. The problem was, as a journalist, I had to be objective. But I found that since I was personally involved, it was difficult and painful. During discussions about the story, glib comments were occasionally made, and I felt very uncomfortable and on the defensive. Also, the people in the photo department thought it would be a good idea to have a photo of a laparoscopy; at that time my wife was about to have one, so they asked me if they could photograph her. Of course they wouldn't use her name or show her face, but I said, "Absolutely not!" I didn't want my wife's stomach in the magazine, especially because everyone there would know it was my wife's stomach. The whole thing was very hard for me to deal with.

Obviously, there is nothing that can be done about mistakes in the past. But you can avoid making further mistakes about your career by trying to separate what you can control in your life and what you can't. Short of finding the best fertility specialists and following their medical advice, there is little you can do about your infertility. However, your career is another matter. That is one important area of your life over which you *can* gain control. According to Dr. Gorman, "It's important to keep intact those aspects of your life that give you a feeling of competence—if you hate your job and feel you are not doing well in that job, then it's important to be active in looking for a job that can give you some personal satisfaction and be a source of strength and comfort."

Turning down good job opportunities because you think you might get pregnant next month can be very self-defeating. You may be setting yourself up for major disappointments in both areas and wind up in a no-win situation. The same is true if you think you are under too much stress to pursue both pregnancy and a new job or new career. Although there are some people like Sue whose doctors' appointments would definitely interfere with a new job, most people can probably successfully make the transition to a new work situation. Says Dr. Gorman, "There are people who turn down job opportunities thinking they can't handle the stress of a new job—meeting new people, dealing with deadlines—so they don't pursue the new job. However, a new and more difficult job sometimes gives you a much greater feeling of success about who you are and what you are capable of doing. Even if you don't feel like doing the work, it can bring you unexpected rewards."

THE FELDMANS

Lisa was working as a secretary in an advertising agency when she first got married, and liked her job very much. She and Eric used to argue about the fact that she wanted to continue working when she had a baby. Even though Eric had just started his private practice and they needed Lisa's income, he felt he didn't want anyone else to raise his child. But instead of getting pregnant, Lisa got promoted and began hating her new position.

LISA: I was never really a career person. My job has never been a very big part of my life. I was very happy as a secretary—I was the best secretary I knew, but, following the "Peter Principle," they kept insisting I was too smart to be doing this, so they kept on moving me up and moved me up until I didn't fit any more. I always liked being an underachiever—it was a lot easier. I've hated this job for a long time now and wanted something else, but I kept thinking it wouldn't be fair to my next employer, since I knew we wanted to get pregnant and I was sure it would happen soon. So I really felt trapped. I was in a state of limbo—no new job, no baby.

ERIC: My career was the most solid base I had—being in medicine, and caring for people. It made me realize that there was something much more important about me than being able to have a good sperm count. I would walk out of that office every day and know that people cared about me.

My career was my solid chopping block, my anchor. It was what I needed, because I was feeling very insecure. It made me identify with my profession, feel good about what I do, but more importantly, it was really something I could lean on.

My retreat was to be constructive and get over the misery and the loss of my dreams of fathering a child. And I realized how fortunate I was having my career—it really made my work very important to me.

If I wasn't dealing with people, I don't know if I could have felt the way I did about not being able to father my own child. That fact, that I was dealing with human lives, probably substantiated the feeling that if I had a child, no matter what the genetic parentage, I would really be an asset to that human life.

Work can be a haven from infertility. It can be a place where you are involved in things and people other than yourself and your problems. It can be a place where your worth is determined by your achievements, not by whether you "pass" a pregnancy test or a sperm test.

Some people find that having a fertility problem helps them reevaluate what can be helpful or rewarding for them and encourages them to seek sources of fulfillment that are more readily available than a hoped-for child.

One of the things that has really surprised me is how much my work meant to me going through this process—how much a support and a lifeline it really became. Before this, I really think if you were to ask me deep inside which was most important, work or family and friends, I would undoubtedly have answered family and friends. What I have found out, because people are the way they are, is that one of the things that has always been there for me is work. And sometimes, when I really would have liked to have stayed home and indulged in being upset, the fact that I had to go teach a class, or write a research grant, or do something that was important to other people professionally, made me feel as if I had a purpose. For me not to do my share would be to inconvenience and cause hardship to a lot of other people. And that sense of responsibility turned out to be a big support.

You don't have to have a professional career in order to gain satisfaction from your work. There are many kinds of jobs that can distract you from your fertility problems and give your life meaning while you pursue parenthood. If you're frustrated because you are not getting pregnant, you can find fulfillment elsewhere. As one woman put it, "I suppose my relooking at the career thing is a lot like feeling that I can't be fulfilled through a child, so I better get my act together about a career." In fact, work of any sort can very much serve as a substitute for a baby, if only temporarily.

> I think ultimately the result of all the frustration and disappointment was that I got more involved in my job. It was a way to try to forget. I worked longer hours; I wanted to be productive. I wanted to produce a baby. I couldn't produce a baby, so I produced a body of work. And I just worked harder and harder. And I was successful. It paid off.

CHAPTER 6

*It's excruciating having to go through this month after month,
having to put your life on such a clinical, systematic chart.
It's terrible having raised expectations and having them
dashed. It's always with me. I wake up with it, I go to sleep
with it, and I think about it literally fifty times a day.
I dream about it. It's night and day, day and night, seven days
a week ever since this began.*

COPING
EMOTIONALLY

THE FELDMANS

Lisa and Eric were discouraged. They knew that unless Eric's
sperm improved, they would have to start seriously looking into
adoption or artificial insemination with donor sperm (AID).
Their second attempt at artificial insemination with Eric's sperm
(AIH) had been a disaster as far as they were concerned, since
there were virtually no sperm in Eric's semen.

> ERIC: It was the most degrading experience. I read the
> counts—it was water!
> LISA: I figured this was God's way of telling us, "OK, it's
> time to adopt." When we spoke to Dr. W., he said, "Lisa,
> you're thirty-four years old. We don't have the time to play
> around. Do you agree?" I agreed. He said he wanted to try a
> few more times with Eric's sperm and if that didn't work, we

would move on to other options, such as adoption or artificial insemination with donor sperm (AID). It wasn't a decision we had to make instantly, because it would be three or four months before a donor would be available. He explained that the AIDS epidemic has made it necessary to screen all donors very carefully each month, thus slowing down the process of donor selection. He then asked us to bring in photographs of ourselves the next time we came.

ERIC: Dr. W. also insisted that in the meantime we go for counseling. He said we could either go to the infertility counselor who worked in his office or to a RESOLVE support group.

I loved the idea because I had been involved with infertility for over a year all on my own, with occasional help from my therapist. It's not that Lisa wasn't involved or supportive, but I couldn't really explain to her what my male feelings were. I never thought I'd be macho about it, but I really was. I always assumed that that would not be a problem with me if I had a fertility problem, that I would want to do the most plausible thing—adopt. I hadn't even considered the possibility of AID. Thank God I had my shrink! My lifelong dream—to have a family—was so important to me for as long as I remember, and now it seemed an impossibility.

The infertility counselor in Dr. W.'s office had a six-month waiting list, so we called the RESOLVE support group leader and set up an appointment. Lisa wasn't particularly interested in going; I had to convince her. I said to her, "Listen, let's go on the interview and see what happens." She said OK. I really wanted to get Lisa involved so she could understand more what was happening to me.

LISA: We met with Beth, the support group leader, and we both liked her, so we decided to try the group. There were four couples altogether—two with male problems and two with female problems. But it turned out all the men actually had fertility problems of one sort or another. We really like one of the couples and became good friends with them, but we sometimes had problems with the other two couples.

ERIC: They never really talked about what they were trying to do—produce families. They were all wrapped up with producing their own biological children. But that wasn't a realistic option for us or for one other couple in which the husband had virtually no sperm.

LISA: The support group was really helpful in that it helped us realize what it was we wanted—a baby. We knew we didn't want to be like some couples who had spent years and years and had nothing to show for it. We wanted a baby and were determined to get one one way or another.

ERIC: My shrink was very supportive of RESOLVE; she felt it was very important for Lisa to go. And she helped me through some really shitty times. She was encouraging me to figure out what I wanted. We talked about Lisa and me having a child first by adoption or AID and then worrying about whether I could father my own child at some future time. It always got back to family.

LISA: My sister and her husband had tried for eighteen years to get pregnant. And I watched it and I lived it. They ultimately did have a baby. But I watched that pain and suffering and I knew I couldn't go through it that long. I always wanted to be a parent with Eric. I decided that it didn't matter a bit whether we adopted, used a donor, or had our own. Eric convinced me to try AID first. He felt strongly that he would rather try AID before we went on to adoption.

ERIC: My feeling was that I wasn't going to be cheated again. I felt cheated that I couldn't have my own child, but I wasn't going to be cheated out of going through a pregnancy with Lisa. It wasn't at all the idea of propagating Lisa's genes. I knew if we adopted I would love the child, but I really wanted to share childbearing.

LISA: It was a very sensitive issue with him, and I felt his feelings on the subject were more important than mine.

ERIC: One night we watched a TV movie about Renée Richards, the doctor/tennis player who changed sexes from a man to a woman. In one scene, years before his sex change operation, he got his girl friend pregnant. I got extremely upset and said, "Even *he* can have a baby!" When I said it, Lisa looked aghast, and we both started to cry.

LISA: Watching Eric's reaction to that movie made me truly understand for the first time what he was feeling. I saw it in his face—it was crystal clear. I really felt his hurt.

ERIC: I had been trying to fight that feeling for a long time
and it was getting me nowhere, just frustrated. But I couldn't
put aside those feelings any more. I had to mourn that
child—we both did. We cried a lot.

SELF-ESTEEM AND SELF-IMAGE

The psychological toll that infertility takes on those experiencing it cannot be overstated. As we have seen in the earlier
chapters, it affects virtually every aspect of one's life—marriage,
sex, work, relationships with family and friends. But infertility
also affects each individual not only in the interpersonal
aspects of their lives, but in a very personal sense as well—
one's self-esteem and self-image.

Sometimes I feel like I have a caricature of a woman's body.
That it's sort of too ripely feminine on the outside and it's no
good on the inside.

My self-esteem has been affected with respect to talking about
infertility with friends who have kids. I feel a self-consciousness
about what they might be thinking—not so much in the sense
that I'm less of a man, but more in the sense that they might
be pitying me.

An important aspect of self-esteem are the feelings of ade-
quacy or inadequacy as a man or woman.

When my husband found out that his motility level was low,
he went into a very deep depression after that. He just really
felt emasculated. He had very big questions about manhood
and all that. And he kept using the word impotent. I kept
saying, "It's not impotence, it's something else." But he kept
using that word. He felt impotent.

It's an ego-battering experience. I don't feel as pretty. I certainly don't feel as fertile or feminine. I feel as though my age
is showing, where I always used to feel I looked younger than
my age, which is thirty-two. I'm really over my prime.

In order to compensate for these feelings, some try to make external changes.

> I started thinking that I was less a woman, less feminine. About that time I started to grow my hair longer. I thought, This must be because I'm feeling unfeminine. Even though I know rationally that being feminine, being a strong female, has nothing to do with these things, here I am doing it. In fact, I stopped wearing loose clothes partly because I didn't want people to think I was pregnant and partly because I decided if I can't be pregnant, goddamn it, I'm going to show off how thin I am! In this stupid country, thinness has such value! And in fact, I did lose weight. I was very thin.

But neither external appearances nor the capacity to bear a child is a true measure of a woman's worth, as one woman finally realized.

> As much as I felt that I shouldn't have the feeling I was a less womanly woman, I did. I went through a period of wanting to look very, very feminine—not wearing pants and letting my hair grow and wearing quite feminine clothes. But I think that I pretty much resolved those feelings. Not being able to have a baby doesn't make me any less womanly than having a baby makes you more womanly; what it is to be a woman is really socially, not biologically, defined.

Nor is the ability to produce sperm that can fertilize an egg a measure of masculinity. In fact, many men *choose* to render themselves permanently sterile by having a vasectomy, and in our society they are usually considered quite "macho." Women also often choose to become sterile by having tubal ligations. Even though these sterile men or women may have had children in the past, they are incapable of doing so in the present, yet they are no less masculine or feminine because of the fertility status.

For men, however, there is no external sign of their fertility or infertility. Infertility does affect feelings of self-esteem in both men and women, but the outward sign of fertility—the pregnant belly—can belong only to the woman. Even if the loss of this capability may be caused by a male fertility problem, it is none-theless primarily the woman who is seen by the outside world as fertile or infertile.

Why Me?

People with fertility problems, like most people when something bad and out of their control happens to them, constantly ask themselves the unanswerable question, "Why is this happening to me? Why can't we do what everyone else does so easily?" When they cannot come up with an answer, some become angry and resentful.

> I was always so careful about contraception—I was the only one of my friends who never had an abortion. Now I'm the only one who doesn't have a baby. Why do I deserve this?

Others look for medical explanations for why they have become infertile. They wind up blaming themselves because they had used an IUD, had VD or an abortion, or delayed childbearing too long. It is true that these things may cause fertility problems in some people, but it's usually impossible to pinpoint the cause. It's also useless to blame yourself; no matter what you had or did, infertility was never your intent. And feeling guilty is not going to help you get pregnant any faster.

Some even develop theories that are totally irrational. One woman told me that she thought she was infertile because she used Q-tips in her ears! And another blamed her vibrator.

> Maybe I never should have used a vibrator. It's not natural; maybe it's too strong an electrical charge and something's happened.

More often, people with fertility problems feel they are being punished for some past deed about which they have lingering guilt feelings.

> I was being punished for wanting to be a career person, for putting things off. I was being punished for being different, for going against my mother's wishes.

I'm Roman Catholic; I used birth control, and maybe this is God's punishment.

Some even feel that God is preventing them from being a parent because they are in some way defective.

Some God or some big computer in the sky or something thinks that there's something wrong with me, either genetically or psychologically or physically, so I'm not to procreate.

Others believe they are not so much being punished as being unfairly singled out to be taught some lesson.

It's as if some sort of divine power has set upon me to have an infertility problem so that I will become compassionate, understanding, sympathetic. But I have done it, I have suffered my sufferings.

I've learned that everything does not always go the way I want it to go. But it seems to me there could have been an easier way for me to learn a lesson like that. I mean, I don't like these big character tests.

And some think they really did learn an important and perhaps necessary lesson.

One of the more philosophical attitudes that I have developed in the last year has been that most people do have a "Why me?" story, and this is my first. I haven't had a parent die or a sibling die or a marriage break up or some terrible disease. There are all sorts of things that people have in their lives. This is mine. Why should I think that nothing's ever going to happen to me—that everything is going to be perfect for us?

There are even those who are able to find a silver lining inside the cloud of infertility, and come to see it almost as a blessing in disguise.

I did have this thing of *Why us? What did we do?* I never had an answer. I just tried to trust that there was a greater reason and a greater scheme of things. We're sort of religious people, and I tried to believe that there was something in the larger picture we didn't see. One of the things, for instance, was that my brother had been sick for so many years, and nobody ever knew where it had come from. And it occurred to me that perhaps there was something genetically wrong, and our not having children was God's way of protecting us from having a severely handicapped child. And the idea came that perhaps my uterus was not strong enough to bear a child, that this was another way God was protecting us from something that was not possible.

What is important is not to dwell on finding an answer to the unanswerable question—*Why me?*—but on the more practical question: What can you do now to resolve your fertility problem both medically and emotionally? An important step in resolving infertility is to accept the situation for what it is, a sad, unfortunate situation that you didn't cause, and to allow yourself to mourn your losses.

LOSS AND GRIEVING

Likewise Lisa and Eric, many couples go through a period of mourning a child they may never have. Grieving is a necessary, if painful, experience that helps the couple come to terms with their infertility, regardless of whether having their own child looks hopeful or hopeless.

According to RESOLVE's Beverly Freeman, "People mistakenly believe that grieving means you're at the end of the road. Grieving can help clear your head and put you in a better position to make decisions about what is best for you, rather than being overwhelmed by the process."

There are a multitude of losses to grieve other than the hoped-for-child—the loss of fertility, the loss of lifelong dreams, and the loss of control over something so fundamental as reproduction. So many losses can lead to depression, especially when one doesn't have the opportunity to grieve.

I have gone through a year of just kind of suffering in silence and making everybody else feel like it didn't matter. And I never really thought about the miscarriage until two years after it happened. After two years it hit me that that might have been my only chance to be pregnant. And nobody let me even talk about it. I never mourned for it.

Unfortunately, many people don't recognize a miscarriage—especially one in the first trimester—for what it is, the death of a potential child. Nor do they recognize a couple's need to mourn a child who never was and may never be conceived.

You really do grieve when you go through this process—when you realize you can't have a child. You must acknowledge that grief to yourself. But the sad part, as a friend of mine pointed out, is it's not as if an actual person has died. So you can't get the kind of support you'd like to get from people because you can't say, "Oh, my mother has died," and everybody knows how to react. This child in me that never existed has died. And you don't know how to say that to people.

According to Miriam Mazor, M.D., clinical professor in psychiatry at Harvard Medical School, "Interestingly, people who handle infertility best are not the first-timers who have never suffered a loss, but those who have suffered losses before, such as the loss of a parent in childhood."

"Grieving is a way to work out feelings so you can gain more control over your life," says Beverly Freeman, "but most people need support in order to help them grieve." That is why support groups can be so helpful; they give couples the permission and opportunity to mourn their many losses with others in the same situation.

THE SPANELLIS

Anthony's sperm count was greatly improved after his varicocelectomy, but Sue had been on Pergonal for seven months with no success. And she still didn't have a diagnosis. They were frustrated, discouraged, angry, and depressed.

SUE: We pretty much realized that there wasn't going to be a pregnancy, so we started going through a mourning process.
ANTHONY: I had been trying to cope by being optimistic

and by denying that we really had a serious problem. I have a tendency not to really acknowledge that a problem exists. If I don't have a problem, I don't need emotional support. So I wasn't getting any emotional support or help from family, friends, or religion, and I was finding it harder and harder to be optimistic. So I went back into therapy. I needed something—I needed not to feel so isolated.

Also, Sue and I were having a real hard time with our relationship at that time. We were both very angry at each other and at our situation and depressed over the whole stupid thing. I kept wondering: Was it worth it?

SUE: I had been on Pergonal for seven months with no pregnancy and was wondering how much of this we could really take. I felt there was some risk of going beyond the limit of what the relationship could take, and not knowing it until we passed that limit. I was so unhappy, and so angry all the time, I really thought we might be better off divorced. At first, dealing with this process of infertility, we used to think it made us closer—that it was a problem we were sharing. But then after a while I started feeling it was detrimental to our relationship. Luckily, we've always been able to talk about things and get them into their proper perspective.

We then took our summer vacation and unknowingly went to a place where there were lots of children. I found that very hard to deal with, and I knew I needed to do something to help me deal with all the emotional issues.

Our only friends with a fertility problem, Judy and Rick, had told us the previous spring about RESOLVE. But I didn't feel like I wanted a support group at that point. However, during that terrible summer, Judy gave me a RESOLVE newsletter and I clipped out the membership form and joined. I was now ready to get involved in a support group.

ANTHONY: I didn't feel the same way. I felt like in a support group, you're just talking about something, but you're not really doing anything medically to help your situation. I said, "Hey, look, we're doing what we have to do medically to get pregnant. Going to a support group and talking about it is not going to make you pregnant." To me, that was the bottom line.

SUE: I really pushed Anthony. It was something I felt that we really needed to do. I felt strongly that it was important to deal with these issues as a couple.

ANTHONY: I finally agreed to go—reluctantly.

SUE: I called the support group coordinator and told her we were interested in a couples' group. She said one was just starting, so we quickly had an interview with the support group leader. We both liked her and decided to try the group, which had already had its first meeting.

I was very nervous going to the group that first time because I wasn't used to talking about this—it felt very risky emotionally to talk about our problems.

There were three other couples with all sorts of fertility problems. They were all very responsive and supportive, especially with regard to the bad experience we had with our first doctor. They all had had similar experiences with bad doctors, and one of the key things we talked about in the group was, Why do reasonably intelligent people continue to go to a doctor for so long when the doctor is obviously not very good?

ANTHONY: It took me a long time to get involved in the group and talk. And when I did talk, I said as little as possible. I like to deal with my problems in my own way. I usually felt antsy and wanted to get out of there.

But the group did help me in the sense that we're not alone. And I kind of liked some of the people there. After a while my feelings changed; I felt it was helping us, and I didn't mind going any more. And I even talked more. I never really liked going, but afterwards I was always glad I had gone.

SUE: It was often difficult for me to talk, but I liked the couples and the group leader, and I knew it was what I needed to be doing even if it was difficult.

One thing that surprised me was how differently people were pursuing medical treatment for infertility. One couple had been trying to get pregnant as long as we had, and they were already well into the process of adoption. They had not really medically pursued pregnancy as comprehensively as we had. But in terms of emotions, a lot of the same feelings were there, and that was reassuring and helpful.

ANTHONY: In a funny sort of way I was glad other people were having these problems too. Except for Judy and Rick, I had never met another infertile person in my life!

SUE: I don't know how I would have gotten through that year of being on Pergonal and having husband inseminations without the support group. That period of time was so difficult for me, I decided to go back and see my old therapist. I was not feeling in control of my life, especially once I started taking Pergonal, because everything was so unpredictable— every month I ovulated at a different estrogen level. One month we discovered after the fact that I had already ovulated before we had a chance to have sex or AIH—that made me very angry, very frustrated, and very dependent on my fertility doctor. I thought my feelings of anger and dependency were something that would more appropriately be dealt with in therapy than in my support group.

My therapist was helpful to me in dealing with the issues of dependency, but I did not find him to be very sophisticated about or sensitive to infertility. The first time I went back to him he said he had some other patients with fertility problems who had been through a lot more than we had! That wasn't what I needed to hear. I mean, I wasn't saying that I had gone through more than anyone else had. What I was saying was that I was in a great deal of pain because of all I had gone through.

He also made several statements to the effect that I should just try to relax, and that made me furious. To me that was basically saying that psychologically I was doing something wrong—I was not relaxed enough to get pregnant. I resented that because I felt like I had done everything I could to get pregnant and was in a situation where it was not going to be easy to be relaxed.

That made me decide to quit therapy, and when I told him why I was quitting, he said what he had meant was that it might help if I was more relaxed *sexually* in terms of getting pregnant! I said to him that that wasn't even relevant to my situation, since I was having artificial inseminations with Anthony's sperm. In any case it was very difficult to be relaxed about trying to get a sperm specimen to the doctor's office and having the sperm-washing done on time and then have to lie there waiting on the examining table to have artificial insemination! So I quit therapy because he wasn't as sensitive to my feelings about infertility as I would have liked.

RELAX AND GET PREGNANT?
ADOPT AND GET PREGNANT?

Perhaps the two things that infertile couples hear the most and hate the most are the phrases, "Just relax and you'll get pregnant," or "Adopt and you'll get pregnant." The implication of both these pieces of advice is that the couple's problem is really psychological, not physical—that the woman herself is to blame for the problem.

It is not only friends and relatives who say or imply this. Unfortunately, many traditional psychotherapists have little understanding about the emotional impact of infertility and even less understanding about the medical issues involved. With female patients, especially, many traditionally trained therapists look for psychological explanations for infertility rather than accept that there might be physiological causes. Yet, unless the infertility is caused by sexual problems such as impotence, therapists are more likely to see male infertility as the result of physical, rather than psychological, problems. They are less likely to suggest to male patients that if they would just relax, they'd be able to impregnate their wives.

Like Sue, many women in therapy are told they are too uptight, too neurotic, or too conflicted about motherhood—and if only they would relax, or get analyzed, they would get pregnant. However, in the majority of cases, there is no evidence of psychological causes of infertility. In fact, in about 95 percent of cases, physical causes can be found. What therapists see—the anger, depression, frustration, low self-esteem, and even ambivalence—are most often the *result* of infertility, not the cause.

According to Machelle Seibel, M.D., associate professor of obstetrics and gynecology at Harvard Medical School, and director of *in vitro* fertilization at Beth Israel Hospital in Boston:

It's the old question, Which comes first, the chicken or the egg? Twenty years ago, about 40 percent of infertility was thought to be caused by emotional factors. Today, with advances in science and technology, a physical cause can be found for infertility in about 95 percent of the cases. The psychological component of infertility is not fully understood, and whether the 5 percent of unexplained infertility is due to psychological causes may never be known.

Dr. Miriam Mazor writes in her book *Infertility: Medical, Emotional and Social Considerations* (Human Sciences Press, 1984):

> The old theories about psychogenic infertility have not only been invalidated, but have generally been counterproductive from both the patients' and therapists' point of view. Patients have avoided contact with psychiatric professionals for fear of being "blamed" or "labeled" pejoratively. Psychotherapy *should not* and *cannot* hold out the promise of pregnancy as its goal. [Emphasis added]

In addition, telling a woman or encouraging her to believe that she is the cause of her own fertility problem does her a great disservice and can only exacerbate any existing psychological problems she may have. Infertility patients often feel guilty enough about their condition without being given one more reason to feel guilty.

> I was recently discussing with my therapist that I see related factors connected with fertility. Sometimes I am willing to believe for myself that the ambivalence is a factor. Or the kind of personality I am. I feel guilty in that very personal way, thinking that there's an emotional connection, a psychological connection, between my own personal self-view and the infertility. It's interesting because there are very real physical things that the doctors can see wrong with both me and my husband.

Suggesting to a couple that if they adopt they will get pregnant also implies that it is the psychological pressure to have a child that is preventing them from conceiving. Again, there is no scientific basis to this assumption. Of course everyone knows couples who adopt and get pregnant. But no one ever mentions their friends or relatives who adopted and *never* got pregnant. You're unlikely to hear someone at a party say, "You know, my friend Karen adopted a baby ten years ago and never got pregnant"—it doesn't make for a very interesting story,

The "adopt and get pregnant" myth is so persistent in this society that medical researchers have investigated it to find out if it is true. Emmet Lamb, M.D., of Stanford University conducted a study on adoption and subsequent pregnancies and concluded that there is no evidence to suggest that infertile women who adopt are more likely to get pregnant than infertile women who do not. On the contrary, he found that the women who adopted were *less* likely to conceive than those who did not adopt. The important thing to remember is that adoption guarantees a baby, *not* a pregnancy. And perhaps you can help dispel the myth by telling people about all the people you know who adopted and did *not* get pregnant.

SOURCES OF EMOTIONAL SUPPORT

Everyone with a fertility problem suffers emotionally—no one is left unscathed. As Dr. Seibel puts it, "Infertile patients are not really sick, just heartsick." Some are more affected than others, and many find that their usual coping mechanisms or support systems are no longer adequate to help them survive the crises of infertility. Often there is an event or turning point that spurs the person to seek outside help.

I had gone down to Atlanta and had spent the whole day in front of TV cameras and on radio talk shows during my so-called glamorous profession, which has seemed a good deal less glamorous ever since I've been trying to get pregnant and haven't been able to. I was traveling back on the plane, and I really thought I was having a breakdown. I started to feel premenstrual symptoms, which to me signified once again that this month didn't work out. Luckily, I was by myself and no one was sitting next to me. I was reading *Glamour* or something to take my mind off my troubles. I was reading frivolous nonsense, and the tears were rolling down. And I was just crying and crying. Two hours from Atlanta to

LaGuardia, and I just spent the whole trip crying. I thought, I'm going to lose my mind. I'm really going to break with reality and go right off the deep end. That was when I decided to call RESOLVE.

Most people who seek emotional help for their infertility problems are really looking for some form of crisis intervention rather than long-term psychotherapy. After all, infertility is a temporary crisis situation. Ultimately there is resolution, and there are various types of emotional support available to help people with fertility problems survive the crisis and resolve their infertility.

There are different resources available to help couples deal with the emotional aspects of infertility.

Traditional Psychotherapists

As long as therapists don't blame the patients for their fertility problems, they certainly can help their patients cope with many of the stresses of infertility. However, most, unless specifically trained, are not really familiar with the medical or emotional aspects of infertility. Just as most gynecologists are not fertility specialists, most psychotherapists are not specialists in dealing with the emotional problems of infertility. According to Roselle Shubin, M.S.W., an infertility counselor in private practice in New York City:

Traditional therapists do not have the biological background to understand the realities of infertility. Infertility is both a crisis situation and an ongoing process as each new test or treatment comes up. The uncertainty presents a crisis, and unless therapists understand the medical aspects of infertility, they can't help the couple understand what the medical issues are and what medical decisions should be made.

In addition, most traditional therapists do not see their role as that of advice givers. If it is practical advice about infertility that you are seeking, you are probably better off looking for an infertility counselor or a support group (see below). If you think you really could use a traditional psychotherapist, you can call your local chapter of RESOLVE; many chapters keep a list of therapists who are interested in and may be sensitive to the issue of infertility—many, in fact, may have had fertility problems themselves. Of course, you are the best judge of whether a therapist is sensitive to your problems and helpful to you.

Infertility Counselors

Some people going through the crisis of infertility may find it helpful to go to an infertility counselor—a psychotherapist who has additional training in reproductive physiology. Infertility counselors can help their patients in different ways than traditional psychotherapists. According to Roselle Shubin, who was trained at the New York University Medical Center:

> An important part of infertility counseling is defining for the couple where they are in the diagnostic workup and treatment process and helping them to know when they are at a point where they should be making decisions and what the implication of those decisions would be. That's not a psychotherapy process. It's more an advisory kind of process like genetic counseling or legal counseling.

Infertility counseling is not an organized profession at present, and the training is not uniform. Says Ms. Shubin, "A lot of people call themselves infertility counselors, and in their minds they may well be doing counseling for the crises that occur around infertility. But for many of them, it's still basically a psychotherapeutic relationship, and that's not what every couple wants or needs."

If you would like to find an infertility counselor, you can call your local chapter of RESOLVE, or you can ask your fertility specialist if he or she can recommend one. Also, an increasing number of medical centers are employing infertility counselors in their departments of reproductive endocrinology or *in vitro* fertilization programs. You can contact the American Fertility Society for information; they are presently compiling a list of such resources.

Again, no matter what your referral source is, you are the only one who can assess if a certain therapist or counselor is appropriate for you and your needs.

Self-Help Organizations and Support Groups

Self-help organizations such as RESOLVE exist in many communities to help couples cope with and resolve their fertility problems. (RESOLVE, the largest organization for infertile couples, has forty-three chapters nationwide.) They also provide practical information on the medical aspects of infertility and such issues as adoption. Other organizations, such as the Endometriosis Foundation, deal with more specific problems. (For a complete list of organizations, see the appendix.)

Most of the local chapters of these organizations have monthly meetings, newsletters, and discussion and support groups. There are in addition many support groups that exist independently of any national organization. In any case, self-help groups provide an excellent opportunity to meet with others with the express purpose of sharing similar experiences and seeking solutions to those problems. For many, it may be the first time they encounter other people with fertility problems.

What was most helpful for me was finding out there are other people similarly situated. I mean, not because misery loves company or to spread the misery around. But at least you know that you have some people to whom you can relate what you are feeling.

Many people, especially men, are resistant to the idea of going to a self-help or support group. However, if they do join, most find that it can be helpful.

My husband Jack's feeling was that if a bunch of us are going to get together and talk about how sad we are that we can't have babies, he didn't want any part of it. So he was very negative. The first time we got together with these people who had fertility problems was when we went to the first meeting of this adoption service where we eventually got our baby. There were about forty couples, all waiting to adopt. Even Jack admitted and agreed that it was the most freeing, most wonderful experience, because it was the first time we talked to anybody about what we were going through. It was the first time we had mentioned to anybody that we had done husband insemination—Jack had been so turned off by it that he didn't want to talk about it with anybody before. It was such a freeing kind of thing, because here were all these other normal, healthy people with nothing deficient about them in any way.

Spiritual Support

Very often people with fertility problems seek help and answers from spiritual sources. As one woman put it, "You look beyond yourself when all else fails." They may or may not have sought spiritual help in the past, but now that they are in a situation that is pretty much out of their control, they turn to religion, the occult, or superstition.

Some find religion and prayer to be a source of emotional support and comfort.

Just recently, I felt that I should try to be more religious, more accepting. I pray a little more, really a little harder. More sincerely. To try to be more accepting of what will be—just accept what God has destined for me, because I can't do any more than I am doing.

I've never prayed for a baby. To this day I've never prayed—you know, lit a candle, done a novena for a baby. I have prayed for strength. God only knows we need a lot of that going through this process. I've prayed for insight to make good decisions for us. In fact, often when I take time off between tests to think about it, it's also to pray about it—is this a good decision for us? Not in a "go to church" kind of way, often just in our own way. I've always felt that there's some sort of master plan guiding your life, and that if we're not meant to do this, we're meant to do something else. And that by making appropriate decisions and being comfortable with them and then moving on to the next step, eventually we will know what it is we're supposed to do.

For some, like one woman who was pregnant again after three miscarriages, religious medals and amulets offer a feeling of protection.

My mother, who is not a religious person, sent me this thing on a chain she got from the television pastor, whom she watches only because my grandmother used to watch. And it says, "Never believe in never." She sent it to me after my first miscarriage. So my impulse was to throw it out. But then I decided to keep it. And I've had it hanging in my room. I just started wearing it a week ago, because I feel I need an amulet.

It's easy to understand how superstitions develop when one feels out of control and afraid.

I was superstitious when I was pregnant, and I violated my superstition that I shouldn't think about the pregnancy or do anything about it. We had gone to this flea market and saw a bassinette. We thought about buying it, and I said no, we shouldn't buy it. But we wound up buying it. And ten days later I had the miscarriage.

Some turn to a combination of religion and superstition to help them get pregnant.

I have a theory that maybe you get pregnant if you're pessimistic rather than optimistic. I've never been a superstitious person, but I've built up so many superstitions about this. It really amazes me, because I always considered myself a very factual person, maybe moral, but never religious and never superstitious. And I became Jewish about this for a while. I thought that if I became Jewish that would help. I was wearing a *chai* around my neck for a year, because that was a symbol of life. I thought if you wore a *chai*, you'd get pregnant. Going to Israel—that was another part of the Jewish year. I made a deal with my husband that if I finished a year of Hebrew lessons, we were going to go on a trip to Israel, because my secret idea was that you go to Israel and you get pregnant. So I went to the land of milk and honey, and my period was five days late. So I knew I was pregnant. Anyway, in the airport coming back, I got my period, of course!

And some believe that fertility symbols may help.

When my wife and I were in Italy on a trip, we bought a small statue in an archeological dig. It turned out to be a fertility goddess. We used to keep it in our living room, but when we discovered we had a fertility problem, we brought it into our bedroom and rubbed it whenever we had intercourse.

DEVELOPING A PERSONAL PHILOSOPHY

Some people are not able to find sufficient help or answers in traditional religion, nontraditional spiritualism, psychotherapy, or support groups. Instead, or in addition, they seek out a personal philosophy to help them survive the crises of infertility.

I probably feel that I have become less religious and more philosophical. In truth it is out of my own hands, and I don't have control over this. Only perhaps by getting information and by making very deliberate and conscious decisions about what I would do next, have I felt that I have some control over it. I think I've come to feel more philosophical about this. And I've gone back and done all kinds of peculiar reading— *The Origin of Species*, *Descent of Man*, *The Meaning of Life*—a lot of philosophy books that I would have hated and did hate as an undergraduate. You know, those kinds of questions have at least for me become very important. And I think I feel kind of together and in harmony with nature, albeit my harmony is in a little bit different key than what most people are going through.

Obviously, whatever works for you to help you cope with and resolve infertility is the best method for you. And you may find that you emerge from the crisis not only with a baby, as most infertile couples do, but with a new perspective on life. As one woman put it, "I've gained an appreciation of what a miracle life is—and pregnancy!"

THE COOPERS

Roy and Mai Li were getting more and more discouraged. Even though she had had extensive surgery for her endometriosis, and danazol treatment for six months after surgery, she had not gotten pregnant. With each passing month their chances for a pregnancy were getting slimmer and slimmer.

ROY: This is not in your control, almost everything else in your life is—you want this thing or you don't want this thing, you can do things to try to attain them. With this, we went as far as we could go—there was nothing we could do. There was no one else to appeal to, no higher authority. If I was religious, maybe I would have gone to a synagogue. Maybe I should have gone anyway.

MAI LI: I even consulted a witch. I went to an office party where they had hired a witch to tell fortunes. This woman was a card-carrying witch, and I consulted her in dead seriousness. I said to her, "I'm trying to get pregnant. Can you help me? Are there any spells, or can you predict what will happen?" And she said to me, "It will happen." Then she told me I had to light a white candle and say a chant, which she gave me. And I did all that! I was willing to try anything!

I was emotionally slipping to the point where I didn't think I could hold up any more. I was too depressed and too terrified and too panicky. I realized I needed help, or I wasn't going to make it. I thought I was going to have a nervous breakdown. I even had thoughts of suicide, because I thought I could not live with this fate.

It was in some ways preposterous or incredible to me that I would be going through this, because I had always gotten everything I wanted in life. Everything always went well; I never had any major illness or death in the family. And it took a really long time to accept the fact that I was really this unlucky. It was a certain feeling of unreality—that I'll wake up from this bad dream someday.

One day I was shopping and a woman came in the store with a newborn baby, and I looked at her and it was like I suddenly lost my sanity. I had this almost irresistible urge to go up to her and say, "Where did you get that baby?" Of course, I knew that she probably gave birth to the baby, but it seemed so impossible. It was impossible for me, who had always been so successful, to do this, that for somebody else to do this seemed like a miracle. I even had fantasies of taking babies, so there were times I was very, very disoriented by my bad fortune. It was grossly unbelievable.

ROY: The predominant feeling for me was sadness. It wasn't so incredible. I didn't dwell on the disbelief of it, it just always came to me and whenever I thought about it, I would get tears in my eyes. It was this overwhelming sadness I never felt before.

MAI LI: I realized that I needed emotional help, and the help I needed would have to be specific to the problem. I found that the general fertile public had difficulty dealing with the depths of my despair; they couldn't relate to it, so I wasn't getting support from them. The other thing that I had was this crushing sense of loneliness that I felt could only be alleviated by being with people like me—people with fertility problems.

So I hit the Yellow Pages and found a fertility clinic listed and called them up and told them I was trying to find a support group or organization for infertile people. They told me about an organization called RESOLVE. I jumped on it and said, "What's RESOLVE?" They told me that it was a self-help organization for infertile couples, and that they had meetings, support groups, and a newsletter. Then they gave me the number of a woman to call. I called immediately and she told me more about the national organization. She told me that they had just formed a local chapter in our area and said, "Our monthly meeting is tonight." I said, "Tonight?" She said, "Would you like to come?" I said, "Absolutely!" I couldn't wait!

ROY: I was really looking forward to going. I felt it was another area of our lives we had to take care of and we were taking care of.

The night of the first RESOLVE meeting I had to give a speech at a big presentation; I was chairperson of a committee of a very large group of cinematographers. There was a whole hoopla, people supporting me and people putting me down, and right in the middle of this, before the important decisions were to be made, I had to say, "Excuse me, I have to go," and I slipped out the back door.

MAI LI: I didn't know if Roy was going to make it. That was just one of those cementing, supportive things where he walked in and I felt this rush of love and feeling connected with him—that we're in this together and he's supportive and I can depend on him. Our relationship really helped me get through this.

I was feeling apprehensive when I went to the first meeting because I didn't know what to expect. I walked in the room, and was struck with how normal people looked. And then I had this secondary feeling that I was part of this secret society. Like aliens. That there was something wrong with everyone there, but they didn't look it. I kept looking at the people to see if their infertility was showing, because I felt so defective.

ROY: I looked around and saw that there were about a dozen people there, and they all seemed bright, educated, and articulate. That really gave me a good feeling, because I saw the potential of this organization was great and we could go somewhere. And all these other people had these fertility problems and were as distressed about it as we were.

MAI LI: I was so relieved finally to be with people like us that I spent the whole time crying. The speaker talked about the emotional aspects of infertility. She started talking about feelings of anger, and it was the first time I acknowledged that I felt angry.

The other thing that I found incredibly sobering was that I hadn't suffered more than anybody else in the world. I was feeling a lot of self-pity and self-righteous rage that I had had to undergo extensive surgery, and nobody else had to do anything like that—it was only me—I was this horrible victim. At the second meeting I went to, we were all sitting around in a circle, and I said, "I had surgery!" And the president said, "Yes, I had it twice!" And this other woman said, "Yeah, I had surgery, too." So it kind of knocked me off my pain pedestal. And I found that helpful.

ROY: I didn't have that same attitude as Mai Li about being the only one who went through this. But there was a general quality about the acknowledgment of the feelings everyone was experiencing. All the cards were on the table; it was all up front.

MAI LI: I was really gung-ho about RESOLVE. The only way not to let this thing get me down was to become really intimate with it. It was really helpful to be involved with RESOLVE. I was even asked to be president of our local chapter, and I said I would be if Roy would agree to be on the board of directors. He did, and I became president.

ROY: RESOLVE itself was a very positive experience for me, and I took the organization very seriously. Besides the usual responsibilities that went with being officers, I arranged for the doctors to speak at our meetings and Mai Li wrote the monthly newsletter. I also wrote reviews of the meetings for the newsletter. We both did a lot of work for the organization—we helped increase the membership of our local chapter from about 50 to 200 in just one year.

MAI LI: I threw myself into RESOLVE work. I tend to embrace situations and be aggressive and enthusiastic about them to try to keep some control over my life, since there was no control with infertility. RESOLVE became very important in my life because it fulfilled a need in me. So I got involved mind, body, and soul.

ROY: RESOLVE became our baby.

CHAPTER 7

*There comes a point in your life when you know you should
stop. I don't know that there are big signals, neon signs
that say, "OK, now is the time." But I think there is a very
subtle sense, "Enough is enough—stop beating your head
against a wall. If it's going to happen, it's going to happen."*

OPTIONS
AND SOLUTIONS

THE SPANELLIS

Sue was now thirty-nine and coming to the realization that if
she hadn't conceived after seven months on Pergonal, her
chances were quite slim. Anthony and Sue frequently found
themselves talking about adoption at home and in their support
group.

ANTHONY: I was getting more and more used to the idea of
adoption, but I would have preferred our own natural child.
What helped me accept adoption more was the support group;
there were two couples who adopted, and that made it much
easier and better. In a way, the decision to adopt was made for
us because we had absolutely no success. I realized that we
could go on like this for ten years and come up empty-handed.
SUE: But one thing that made the decision to move toward

adoption more complicated was that we had no diagnosed problem, since Anthony now had a good sperm count. I think it's easier if you know your odds are very slight or nil. But when you go through years without a diagnosed problem, it's very difficult to know when to say we'll move on to adoption and stop, or move on to adoption and keep trying—that was difficult for us.

ANTHONY: We had previously gotten a lot of information about adoption from RESOLVE and the Adoptive Parents Committee and realized that we were probably too old to be accepted by an adoption agency. Also we found out that with private adoption, you can get a newborn infant, but babies from agencies are first placed in foster care for several months before they can be adopted.

We got the name of our friends' adoption lawyer and went to see him. He saw five couples at once and went through all the general procedures about private adoption—what to be aware of, what to do, what not to do, what to say, what not to say, how to put ads in small-town newspapers and install a private phone with an unlisted number so we could be contacted by the pregnant women. He then saw each couple separately to answer specific questions. I thought he was competent and could do the job.

SUE: I was depressed after that meeting; he was very realistic about how it could be a long, complicated process. Intellectually we knew that, but we also knew several couples who had been very lucky and adopted newborn babies within a few months of trying to adopt.

ANTHONY: The one thing that really bothered me was the procedure; I did not like the idea of advertising in a newspaper for a baby. It seemed so crass. That's *not* how we thought we'd get a baby.

SUE: We also got information about international adoption and Jerry Falwell's group, Save a Baby, but that group said we would have to become "born again Christians" and that was definitely *not* part of our plans!

By the summer, we had not had a break from trying to get pregnant in over three and a half years. We decided it was time to have another consultation with Dr. P.

We told him we needed a break, that we wanted to take a month off. And we also told him that we were really going to start seriously exploring adoption now, try Pergonal for another three months and then give up. Dr. P. said that sometimes before a couple stopped medical treatment he liked to have the woman have a second-look laparoscopy as a final check.

Our feeling was that if he was going to do another laparoscopy after three more months on Pergonal, why not do it before? And if there was something wrong—although we couldn't believe that there would be, since our first doctor hadn't found anything significant during the first laparoscopy two years before—why not have it diagnosed before we go through three more horrible months of Pergonal and inseminations? My doctor thought that was a good idea and told me that since he no longer did surgery, the head of the clinic would do it. I decided to have it done.

The surgeon found adhesions on my tubes and cysts on my ovaries and a large cyst at the end of my tubes—any of which could have prevented me from getting pregnant! And my previous doctor hadn't found anything wrong!

Before surgery I had given permission for more extensive surgery if necessary, so the surgeon removed the cysts and adhesions. So I had my surgery—a little more than I expected! Dr. P. and the whole staff were amazed that they found these things wrong with me. Anthony and I were both very angry—all that time and all those drugs and inseminations had been wasted.

ANTHONY: I was really annoyed with our first doctor, and with the fact that we trusted her and her laparoscopy report. Why couldn't we have done this sooner?

SUE: I was *very* depressed at the thought that I already had gone through so much that turned out to have had little likelihood of working. I felt terrible. I lay there in the hospital after that, feeling very poorly physically and really depressed, and I kept thinking, if I had known what these last several years would be like before we ever even started to try to get pregnant, I would have just said, let's adopt. I just lay there and thought, God! What a horrible year!

And to make matters worse, when I got home, I had an infection from the incision and was in a lot of pain. Then on top of that, I had an allergic reaction to either the pain medication or the antibiotics. It was *just horrible*!

My husband and my doctor, on the other hand, were excited because something had been found. In fact, while I was recovering, Anthony went to our support group alone, and he was so excited everyone was certain that I was pregnant!

ANTHONY: I felt very good. I thought, this just may very well be it! After three and a half years, we finally found out what it was that was wrong. I felt very, very hopeful.

SUE: I asked the surgeon what my chances of conceiving were now that he had removed the adhesions and cysts. He said that without taking other things into consideration, such as my age and Anthony's condition, the prognosis seemed very good. I was glad to hear that, but it was hard for me to believe by that time that I might possibly be able to get pregnant.

A month and a half after surgery, Dr. P. wanted to start me on Pergonal again. Since I now had a diagnosis, we weren't quite ready to quit just yet. So we decided to go ahead with the original plan and try for three more months on Pergonal and AIH. However, it was becoming very difficult emotionally to keep doing all this medical stuff.

I was forcing myself to keep going on, cycle after cycle, with no results. We decided that we had better start working on adoption again if we ever wanted to have a child.

ANTHONY: We wanted to see another lawyer so we would have a choice. The second one we went to, a woman, was warmer, but both lawyers we interviewed seemed equally competent.

SUE: We felt good after the meeting with her and positive about her, but she was talking about more money. Her adoptions averaged $11,000 or $12,000 and his $7,000 to $8,000.

ANTHONY: I agreed to go ahead and place the ads in the newspaper, though I still didn't like the idea.

SUE: In December, we brought our extra phone down from our country house and arranged to have the phone installed after we got back from our winter vacation.

That month we had the worst cycle we had yet, in terms of my hormones being out of synch with the Pergonal. It just wasn't working.

ANTHONY: I was beginning to get myself emotionally ready to go through the adoption routine. I was resigned.

SUE: I got very excited about the prospect of adoption. By then we knew several couples who adopted, and their children were wonderful.

I was also very concerned about my age; I was almost forty! I felt that if I wanted to have a child it was enough time already. We had gone on long enough.

January was going to be our last cycle on Pergonal. I was *very* anxious. It looked like my hormones were once again out of synch. I called Dr. P. on Friday evening. He suggested that we should take a few extra days of Pergonal over the weekend and have intercourse in case I hadn't yet ovulated. On Monday I had some more blood tests so we could know when to do the insemination. When I called Dr. P. that afternoon, he said it looked like I had already ovulated, so it wasn't worth coming in for AIH. It had been our last chance. It was a difficult time for us.

ANTHONY: I was disappointed once again.

SUE: Two weeks later I felt premenstrual—I started to feel crampy and depressed, so I took my cramp pills. But my period didn't start. I was sure that the lab had made a mistake about when I ovulated, so my period wasn't really late. I was terrified to believe that I could be pregnant. I felt like I would be *so* devastated if I let myself be really hopeful and then found out that I wasn't pregnant.

ANTHONY: We decided not to get our hopes up too high because we knew of somebody in our support group who was ten days late, and it turned out she wasn't pregnant.

SUE: We waited until my period was a week late before calling Dr. P. He was very guarded, but he did suggest that I come in for a pregnancy test. So I went in. I felt very nervous. And I kept feeling like I was about to get my period.

They said the results would be ready at four o'clock. I waited nervously all day. I told Anthony to be by this phone at four sharp.

ANTHONY: I didn't want to get my hopes up, so I didn't think about it all day.

SUE: I called my doctor at four and got disconnected! I was a nervous wreck! I called again and finally got through and Dr. P. said, "You are *definitely* pregnant!" I said, "Really, I can't believe it! Is that test ever wrong?" He said, "Not in my experience." I said, "That's amazing!" He was very excited, too.

I called up Anthony. The phone rang a few times and I thought, God, where is he? Why isn't he sitting right by the phone waiting to grab it immediately? He finally answered and I said, "I'm calling you to tell you your wife is pregnant."

ANTHONY: I was ecstatic!

SUE: I tried to call my sister, but her line was busy. So I went out and bought a bottle of champagne to share with the people in my office—they had all been so wonderfully supportive. When I got home, Anthony had a bottle of champagne waiting. We celebrated and called our families. I'll never forget how Anthony told his mother. He called her up and said, "*Eh Ma! Sue es gravida*"—Sue is pregnant!

WHEN ENOUGH IS ENOUGH: EXPLORING OTHER OPTIONS

Like Anthony and Sue, about half the couples who seek treatment for infertility give birth to a child that is genetically related to them both. They may have conceived with the help of drugs and surgery, as Anthony and Sue did, or with the help of some of the new reproductive technologies, such as *in vitro* fertilization.

But although having a baby that is genetically related to *both* the husband and the wife may be the optimal outcome, it is unrealistic and unlikely for many infertile couples. There are other genetic options that allow the couple to have a child that is related to the wife (by donor sperm) or the husband (by surrogate motherhood). For many, these options are unavailable or unappealing, and they opt to have a child that is not genetically related to either one, and adopt a baby.

Before any options are considered, however, the couple, if

they really want to have a child, must be able to accept the idea that their pursuit of pregnancy may have to be replaced by a pursuit of parenthood. Getting to that point is not always easy. First, they must both accept the fact that it's not going to happen in the way they had hoped. Then they must ask themselves whether they can love a child that is not genetically related to them. And finally, they must both agree about what should be done next.

According to RESOLVE's Beverly Freeman, "There may be disagreement as to what to do next. It may be time for them to stop, at least temporarily, to check in with each other and make sure that they are both doing what they want to do. They may be ready to stop, to proceed with adoption, or to find some other option that is best for them, including child-free living." Also, by stopping and reevaluating the situation, the couple can often set reasonable goals for how much longer to continue pursuing pregnancy, if that is what they wish.

Not all of these options are desirable or even appropriate for each couple, but they all represent the same thing to the couple—giving up the dream to have a child that is biologically related to them both. This is very difficult for most couples to do, because most of us grow up thinking that the genetic bond is the strongest and most important. In addition, most dream about having a child with their looks and other family traits such as intelligence and artistic or athletic ability. Of course, most don't stop to think about some of the negative family traits that can be passed on, such as genetic predisposition to certain mental and physical diseases.

Also, according to infertility counselor Roselle Shubin, another reason couples find it so difficult to say enough is enough is that "psychologically you rebel against the concept that something you wanted so much and tried so hard to achieve will not happen. And some people think that stopping means they are quitters. They can't see the difference between quitting and accepting reality."

Deciding "enough is enough" is usually a gradual process, unless one has a doctor who says, "There is nothing more to be done medically." However, most doctors don't like to be so absolute in their pronouncements. According to Ms. Shubin:

There are couples who have pursued pregnancy for many years at the expense of so much else in their lives, and no one has been kind enough to say, "Stop, it probably will never happen." But medical people almost never use the word "never," and that's the phrase many people are waiting to hear. The couple often has to decipher what the doctor means when he says, "Things don't look good, but of course there's always a chance."

One thing you and your spouse can do is meet with your doctor and ask more specifically what your odds for conceiving are, and how long it might take. You should also ask him if he can recommend another treatment method that he might not be equipped to do, such as *in vitro* fertilization. You then have to take into account such personal factors as your age, finances, and ability to tolerate more treatment as well as the all-important question of what is it you *really* desire, pregnancy or parenthood. No doctor can answer those questions for you. As one woman put it, "At one point I didn't really know if it was the desire to have a child that was driving me or the desire to finally succeed."

For those of you who are still actively pursuing pregnancy and are not sure if you are ready to pursue other options, there are some clues you can look for, according to Diane Clapp, B.S.N., R.N., medical information counselor at National RESOLVE. It may be time to stop trying and pursue other options

- if you find that you are fantasizing more about adoption or child-free living, and/or more of the books on your bedside table are about these options than about infertility.
- if you compare how you felt about an option such as AID or adoption when you first started infertility treatment with how you feel about it now, and find that the option has moved from "second best" or "out of the question" to "not such a bad idea after all."
- if previously you were excited by the prospect of a doctor's appointment or new treatment and now feel oppressed, depressed, and exhausted by that prospect or by the medical processes in general.

- if you can imagine your doctor saying to you, "I'm very sorry, but there is nothing more that I or anyone else can do to help you," and you feel more relief than panic.

If you do decide that it is time to stop trying and pursue other options, then you must decide whether you are more interested in a *genetic* option, such as surrogate motherhood or AID, or a *nongenetic* option, such as adoption or even child-free living. What is most important is that both spouses agree on what option they will pursue next. Let's look more closely at some of these options.

GENETIC OPTIONS

Surrogate Motherhood

One of the most widely publicized and controversial of the genetic options is surrogate motherhood, and not without good reason. Unlike AID, in which a donor provides the sperm to produce a child and never has anything further to do with the mother or child, in surrogate motherhood a woman is chosen by the infertile couple, is artificially inseminated with the sperm of the prospective father, and, if she conceives, carries the child to full term. She is usually paid a fee, typically $10,000 if she is not a friend or relative. Theoretically, after the child is born, the woman gives it up for adoption to the infertile couple. There are, however, potential problems.

Surrogate motherhood involves the physical, legal, ethical, emotional, and often financial commitments of the biological mother. The natural result is that some surrogate mothers, when the time comes to relinquish the baby, find that they cannot go through with it. This recently happened in New Jersey in the much-publicized case of Baby M, in which a surrogate mother sued for custody of the child she bore for another couple. (She lost.) At present, the legal status of surrogate motherhood is uncertain; there are no laws protecting either the couple who contract for a surrogate mother or the surrogate mother herself.

Infertile couples not only get to choose the biological mother *before* pregnancy but, in some instances, have frequent contact with her during pregnancy, especially if she is a friend or relative, and in some cases are even with her at the delivery. Close contact with the surrogate mother is no guarantee that she will relinquish her baby, however, and even if she does, the emotional effects of this involvement between surrogate mothers, infertile couples, and resulting children can cause a great deal of stress and confusion. According to Roselle Shubin,

It's not just the legalities couples should be warned about. Couples are putting an awful amount of love and an awful amount of money into a situation where neither they nor anybody else can predict how the biological mother will feel once she has gone through the birth experience. The infertile couple is already at a point where they have used up their emotional energy and are very vulnerable. To go through such an uncertain situation at that point can be extremely dangerous for a couple.

Another potential problem is that the surrogate mother must be trusted to abstain from sexual intercourse for long periods while she is being artificially inseminated; otherwise, paternity could be in doubt. This has happened in several cases where the child born was not in fact fathered by the donor, but by the husband or boyfriend of the surrogate mother.

Surrogate motherhood raises many yet unanswered legal, social, and ethical problems. For this reason, both RESOLVE and the American Fertility Society (although they agree that there is a legitimate need for surrogate motherhood) do not fully endorse the practice at this time. According to the most recent American Fertility Society ethical guidelines, published in its medical journal, *Fertility and Sterility* (Vol. 46, No. 3, Supp. 1, September 1986):

The [Ethics] Committee does not recommend widespread clinical application of surrogate motherhood at this time. Because of the legal risks, ethical concerns, and potential physical and psychological effects of surrogate motherhood, it would seem more problematic than most of the other reproductive technologies discussed in this report. The Committee believes that there are not adequate reasons to recommend legal prohibition of surrogate motherhood, but the Committee has serious ethical reservations about surrogacy that cannot be fully resolved until appropriate data are available for assessment of the risks and possible benefits of this alternative. The Committee recommends that if surrogate motherhood is pursued, it should be pursued as a clinical experiment.

Any couple considering this option should make certain they understand all the risks involved. You should read as much as you can (see the suggested reading list at the end of this book) and, if possible, discuss this option with a fertility counselor or support group. Of course you should find a surrogate through a legitimate source and make certain she has been carefully screened both medically and psychologically. And, last but not least, make certain you have a good lawyer who is experienced in drawing up legal contracts with surrogate mothers.

Artificial Insemination by Donor (AID)

This is a more socially and legally accepted, as well as widely used, genetic option for the infertile couple with male infertility as the primary problem. It has been estimated that at least 10,000 AID babies are born each year in the U.S.

In AID the husband must relinquish his dream to father a child, whereas the wife is able to fulfill her dream to conceive and give birth to her own child. It is often a more difficult decision for the husband, since he is the one who won't have any genetic input into the child. But it's important to remember that in *every other* sense he will be the child's father. In fact, there has never been a case where the donor has been held legally responsible for an AID child. The California Supreme Court decided in 1968: "The anonymous donor of the sperm cannot be considered the 'natural father,' as he is no more responsible for the use made of his sperm than is the donor of blood or a kidney." According to Sherman J. Silber, M.D., a urologist and reproductive microsurgeon at St. Luke's hospital in St. Louis, Missouri:

There should be no ethical, moral, or legal question as to who is the father. The father, according to most laws and most books, is the man living with the woman who bears the child. The donor has no social relationship at all to the child—he just provided some sperm. The donor has no feeling whatsoever for or identification with the child.

In addition, Dr. Silber points out that it's important to remember that in the "nature versus nurture" debate, nurture very often comes out the winner—intellectual accomplishments, personality, and even athletic ability are often more the product of the child's environment than his or her genes. For those who are excessively concerned about intelligence, most donors are carefully screened medical or law students. (That may not, however, be reassuring to everybody!)

Some even see advantages in having children who are *not* genetically related to them because of fear of passing on some undesirable family traits.

For me, and it's been a gradual process in coming to terms with this, the thing that is really important is to raise a child. And it *isn't* the most important thing that the child be physiologically mine. In fact, I've been thinking of some of the advantages for it not to be mine—I wouldn't be responsible for its defects. I've always favored the idea of having a boy, and this, I'm sure, is a common male response, but one of the main reasons is the desire to do right the things my father did wrong. And by having a child that is not biologically mine, I'd be halfway there already!

Dr. Silber, who is also the author of a book on infertility, *How to Get Pregnant* (Warner Books, 1981), advises,

AID should only be embarked upon when (1) you know that that is what's necessary—that without AID the wife cannot conceive; and (2) you are sure you are making a rational decision that you can live with 'til the end of your days—that you won't mind that the kid has another man's genes.

Donor insemination, when the wife has no fertility problem, is as successful as natural conception—that is, each month the woman has a 20 percent chance of conceiving. With repeated cycles, the overall pregnancy rate for couples undergoing AID is 80 to 90 percent, according to Dr. Silber. AID is also cheaper than adoption, and, unlike in adoption, the couples get to share the pregnancy and childbirth experience. However, it is definitely *not* for every couple. Many couples feel strongly that if they can't have a child that is genetically related to both of them, then they would rather adopt than do AID. Others have very strong emotional reactions to the very idea of donor sperm. In addition, some religions such as Roman Catholicism and Orthodox Judaism are opposed to AID.

There is some controversy as to how couples who have undergone this procedure do in the long run. Certainly, just as some biological parents and adoptive parents split up, some couples who have undergone AID also split up. Says Dr. Silber,

> From my experience and the experience of most of my colleagues, I think it's very clear that the vast majority of AID couples who succeed are delighted with what they have done. In fact, many not only want another AID baby, but the same donor.
>
> And in my experience, the divorce rate in these couples is very low—lower than in the general population. I think the reason is that in general, it requires a tremendous ability to communicate rationally in the face of a difficult emotional situation to come to the decision to have AID. And for the most part, couples don't embark upon AID unless they've really got a quality relationship.

There are, however, many potential social and psychological problems concerning AID, and every couple considering this option should be aware of them. For example, many husbands of women having AID become temporarily impotent, perhaps because they unconsciously feel their wives have been unfaithful. Couples will also have to face the issue of whether to tell anybody, including the child, that an anonymous donor is the genetic father.

Therefore, before making a decision, any couple seriously considering AID should, if possible, consult an infertility counselor or join a support group to discuss further the pros and cons of this option. Furthermore, the couple would be well advised to do as much reading as they can on the subject (see appendix).

Lori B. Andrews, J.D., an attorney specializing in the new reproductive technologies, writes in her book *New Conceptions* (St. Martins Press, 1984):

> If both husband and wife have been open about their feelings about AID and come to terms with their emotions, the pregnancy can be a stunningly happy time for them. The satisfaction that most couples ultimately feel about the baby born to them through AID is reflected by their willingness to undergo the process again. Ninety-eight percent of those couples who bear a child via AID feel their decision was the right one and a majority of those who have AID children decide to have another child in the same manner.

THE FELDMANS

Although Eric's sperm sample had been very poor when they did their last husband insemination, they decided to keep trying AIH until a donor was found for them. Dr. W. had told Lisa at her last appointment that it would probably take three or four months before an appropriate donor could be found.

LISA: A few days after I saw Dr. W., I got a phone call at work from his nurse, Vicky. She said, "We have a donor for you." Only a few days before, they said they would have a donor in three or four months! I was shaking. I said, "Book me!" I figured I could always cancel. I called Eric and all he could say was, "Oh, my God! Oh, my God!"

ERIC: I couldn't believe it—all of a sudden a phone call— guess what? Bingo! Superstar is here!

When we got home, we each poured a glass of wine and sat down and talked. Lisa looked at me and said, "What do you want to do?" I said, "Not now! I'm not ready for it." It was too premature; we had just started to talk about this. We thought we had at least four months to think about it and to try some more with me. Lisa said if I still wanted to try it some more with my sperm, that would be OK—she'd do that first.

But I knew we would ultimately do it, so in a sense I was ready; I just needed more time. I believed Dr. W., and I had done a little research. I had looked at the counts; I knew what motility really meant, it wasn't just a word, and I didn't have much of a chance. My motility and concentration were bad. I kept thinking, we can do this *now!* And I knew Lisa probably wouldn't get pregnant the first shot anyway, so there would be time to try me again.

It really wasn't a big decision for us, because we thought we had done all the field work we could—we went for consultations, we went for therapy, we reached a point where Lisa said, "Eric, what do you want and how important is it that the kid looks like you?"

LISA: I was convinced to try AID because Eric's feelings were much more important than mine at this point, since it was a very sensitive issue with him. He felt strongly that he would rather do AID than adopt.

So we decided to go ahead. I made an appointment for the following Saturday, when I was supposed to ovulate. A few days before the insemination I absolutely freaked. The idea of foreign sperm was *so* disgusting. And I screamed at Eric, "How could you want me to do this?" My worst fantasy was that it was like *Rosemary's Baby*. Then I found out when I went to our support group that this feeling passes. Two other women who had AID had the same reaction, and it passes. I began to think of the donor sperm as medicine, and it clicked. I said, OK, if it's medicine, it's all right.

The other thing I realized is that *any* sperm would be foreign to me. Whether it was from my husband or a stranger, it was from another being.

ERIC: I thought more about it in the next few days waiting for Lisa to ovulate. I really wished we had more time, but there was a part of me that wanted out of that whole scene. I don't know how long I could have done it in a jar every month.

LISA: I woke up Saturday morning and was very excited. I kept thinking, oh, boy, it's my turn now—now I can do something. Eric had been the one working at it up 'til now.

ERIC: I was nervous as hell when we got to the office. When I'm nervous, I get hyper. I was talking very loud and cracking jokes.

LISA: Eric's a performer. There was only one other woman

in the waiting room, obviously another AID since it was Saturday, and Dr. W. wasn't in. The nurse, Vicky, was going to do the insemination. We waited and waited and finally Vicky came out and said, "I'm afraid that there's been a delay; the messenger was late picking up the sperm."

ERIC: I went into her office. She said it shouldn't be much longer; she seemed very nervous and made some phone calls and lots of excuses. Then she said, "I'm going to the hospital now to pick it up. Just wait here and please answer the phone for me."

LISA: When Vicky came back she just walked into her office without saying whether she had the sperm or not. She came out a few minutes later. She was frantic and said, "He's still not here! But he should be here very shortly—can you wait?" We said, "Of course." While she was in the back office, the front door buzzer rang, and since there was nobody to answer the door Eric got up and opened the door.

ERIC: Vicky came running out and *pushed* me aside and led the man who was at the door into the hallway. All I could see was the man's back. He didn't look like a messenger, but it didn't occur to me that he might be the donor!

LISA: I saw him from the back and said to Eric, "That's not a messenger, that's him!"

ERIC: I heard him talk to Vicky and apologize for being late and knew for sure it was him. I thought, My God! Here is the man who is giving the sperm that might get my wife pregnant!

LISA: I wanted to get a good look at him to make sure he wasn't a fat slob or anything, but Eric kept pushing my face away and said, "Don't look, it's not important!" I yelled at Eric, "Get out of my way!" because he was leaving and I wanted to get a good look to make sure he was a "regular person."

As he was leaving I was able to see him for a second. He was thin and had a mustache like Eric, which I liked. He also had brown, curly hair and was about Eric's height. And he was well dressed in a nice overcoat. He looked like a normal person. That was *so* important to me. That's all I wanted to know—it satisfied everything I needed to know. I mean, if he was a fat shlep, I wouldn't have done it.

ERIC: I went into the examining room with Lisa. Here was my wife, about to be inseminated by a stranger! I really got a little bit misty—and then, a little bit crazy.

LISA: I got undressed and got up on the examining table and Eric sat by my side holding my hand, just like he did whenever I had AIH. But this time his hand was sweaty. Vicky walked in and said, "I just looked at the donor's sperm under that microscope, and this guy is a stud!" That's when Eric freaked.

ERIC: Yeah, I really felt good then. All the time I was sitting there I had been thinking there was hope for me—that my sperm would improve so *I* would be able to impregnate my own wife.

LISA: Vicky then said, "OK, here we go," and Eric turned absolutely white and started shaking.

ERIC: I started to cry. I had a very difficult time with the thought of somebody going into my wife's body that wasn't me. That was my macho part again—I wasn't able to make Lisa pregnant, so I felt like a failure. but I was also crying about all the energy that went into this—a year-and-a-half's worth—and here was somebody who was going to stick in a syringe with somebody else's sperm! And here I was in the room holding my wife, and she was trying to get pregnant and it wasn't me! I really felt the loss right there.

Vicky was wonderful, very supportive. She told me that another husband had reacted just the same way I did. She made me feel better. She said, "It's always very difficult. I know you're a nice man and you'll be a wonderful father, and all I can tell you is that somehow down the road, if things do work out, when you hold that child in your arms all this won't be important—it will all disappear." By then, I was whimpering. It made me feel better; she gave me tissues. But it was everything—it was my life. The problem was having to deal with it *now*.

LISA: When it was over, we went out and had brunch at a deli and soothed our pains.

ERIC: We both had chicken soup!

LISA: When we got back home, I felt very, very special. I felt wonderful. I guess I wasn't hooked into Eric's feelings.

ERIC: I wasn't feeling so wonderful. I felt weird because I felt the noninvolvement part—that I wasn't there. But I kept thinking that I really *was* there, and I kept thinking about what we were doing this for. Lisa and I felt very close afterwards. I was very sure that I was going to deliver *my* sample that night. And I did.

LISA: Eric's sister and her lover, who were still trying to get pregnant with AID, told us that they heard that it helped to have an orgasm after inseminations.

ERIC: Also, it gave me some sort of out if she did become pregnant—that maybe it would be me after all.

I felt overwhelmed because the insemination happened so fast. And I felt angry that I couldn't be a part of it. It wasn't easy. I didn't feel great. I didn't feel ready to go dancing.

LISA: I was worried about Eric. He was a mess. When I made an appointment for another donor insemination two days later, Vicky suggested that I leave Eric home. Eric and I were both relieved. It was much easier the second time without him.

ERIC: I spoke to Lisa on the phone after the second insemination and I said, "How was it? Did you see him again?" You know, the normal jokes. She told me that it went very smoothly and that Dr. W., who did the insemination this time, said she was definitely ovulating. He also apologized to Lisa for what had happened on Saturday. He said it had *never* happened before and would *never* happen again. By Wednesday, I started to feel better about the whole thing.

LISA: What we kept saying over and over was that we learned to love our ASPCA cat—that it feels like ours. So we knew we would be able to love our AID baby—it would be much easier.

I had asked Dr. W. if anyone ever gets pregnant the first month. And he said, "Hardly ever." I asked how long it might take and he said, "You'll have to allow four to six months." We've always been very pragmatic and set goals. I felt we had to put a lid on it, so I decided that I would try AID for one year and if I didn't get pregnant we would adopt.

After the second insemination, Eric started having fantasies about me having been unfaithful. I didn't find out about it until a week later at our support group. It just slipped out—Eric said something about me having sex with another man. And Beth, our support group leader, said, "Eric, did you hear what you just said?"

ERIC: I didn't really feel that she was unfaithful. I was really feeling that somebody was penetrating my wife without me having anything to say about it. But I *did* have something to say about it. That was jive—it was just me trying to accept it.

LISA: My periods are always very regular and two weeks after Dr. W. said I had ovulated, Monday morning, I didn't wake up with my period. I was doing my Jane Fonda exercises that evening, as always, and when I got to the end, I blacked out. It was like a black cloth was over my eyes. I stopped and said to Eric, "Something's wrong. I know I'm pregnant." And he said, "No, you're not, that's ridiculous!" The next day I called my doctor's office and told them I blacked out while exercising and hadn't got my period yet. They said, "Get in here for a blood test!" I said, "You're kidding—it's only three days late!" At this point, I was furious at Eric because he wouldn't talk to me about it at all.

ERIC: I kept on saying that it couldn't be. Dr. W. had said it hardly ever works the first time. In a way, I was hoping that it couldn't be. In my heart, I was hoping that there still was a chance for me. This donor was just a fly-by-night.

LISA: I tried to talk to Eric again on Tuesday night, and he still wouldn't talk about it. I was pissed off, so on Wednesday I went by myself for the blood test and didn't tell Eric I was going. Vicky said to call for the results the next day at three o'clock.

The next morning Eric leaned over in bed and asked me if I got my period, and I said no. He said, "OK, you can go for your blood test today." I said, "Well, thank you!"

ERIC: Lisa then said, "Do you want to know a secret?" And she showed me the bandage on her arm. By now I was excited, but I didn't think there really was a chance. It never happens the first time. My sister had been trying AID for two years and still wasn't pregnant. Also, I couldn't believe that after I couldn't do it in over two years, this guy could do it in two "beef-jerky" injections!

LISA: We had to wait until three that afternoon. The waiting was horrible. At five to three I couldn't wait any more. I called Vicky and she said, "Congratulations!" I said, "WHAT?" And I burst into tears. I was on the phone in the hall at work crying hysterically. I hung up and called Eric.

ERIC: Lisa called me at the office, and I was surrounded by people. When I answered the phone, she said, "Congratulations!" The whole world stopped. I just sat there and froze and then cried. I was so happy, I didn't stop grinning for a week!

Lisa's pregnancy progressed normally. And neither of them seemed to have any trouble accepting the fact that Eric was not the biological father. Lisa had amniocentesis, and the fetus was healthy. They chose not to know the sex.

LISA: After the amnio, Eric kept saying, "I hope it looks like you."

ERIC: I think seeing the fetus during the amniocentesis stirred up all these old feelings I can't put aside. I'm allowed to be sad. I can mourn that child—I still have hope for that child some day, being "subfertile." We're going to try again.

LISA: But in the meantime, we're about to have what we really wanted.

ERIC: Absolutely, there's no question about it, we need a family. And the genetic hookup is really irrelevant. The only time I think of it as not being my child is when I see a father with a child who looks exactly like him. I asked Lisa, "Do you envision what this child is going to look like? Has it been a major concern of yours?" She said no.

I see fathers and daughters or fathers and sons and I see that genetic hookup and I say, "There's this mystery now." I hope it looks like Lisa because that's a base I can identify with. And Lisa has some outstanding characteristics that are in her family—the jet-black hair and emerald-green eyes. I hope I have that identity; it would make it easier. Of course it still affects me. Of course I'm still wondering what the child will look like.

LISA: The times Eric sees those children looking exactly

like the father or mother, what he doesn't see is that they look *nothing* like the other parent. When he points to a child that looks just like the father I say, "But look at the mother, the child looks nothing like her!"

ERIC: Lisa said that the most important thing, as crazy as it sounds, is, "Now we'll have someone to say Kaddish [the Jewish prayer for the dead] for us when we die." I said, "Wow! *That's* a real special person!" The Jewish traditions are very important to me.

LISA: When I was in my sixth month, a friend was planning a bris [circumcision ceremony] and asked me some questions about it. I had this book called *The Second Jewish Book of Why's*, so I said, "I'll look it up." It's a fascinating book. I started to read it, and I came across this section on infertility and saw this question about why Jews didn't believe in donor insemination. I had never heard that before. I said to myself, "I don't want to know this," and I put the book down. Eric said, "What were you reading?" and I said, "Oh, just something about brises."

ERIC: I picked up the book and started to leaf through it. And the first page I opened up to was the page on AID. The first question was on why AIH was basically OK. The second question was, "Why does AID exist and how do we look upon it?" And what it basically said was that the child was a bastard, and that I was creating a sin by allowing it to happen to my wife, who was considered a whore by accepting the donor's sperm!

I'm sitting there reading this and I'm getting this schizo kind of feeling in my head and I thought, This doesn't make sense. My body's changing and I'm feeling like something was churning in my heart. I said to Lisa, "Listen, I really have to get some sleep." And what I did was I went inside and thought. I was trying to figure it all out. This was breaking a basic bond I had with my religion all my life. I was a sinner, my wife was a whore, and I was going to raise a bastard! Other than that, I was having a great time!

The only thing that kept me clear was thinking, How could anyone who could preach holiness, which is goodness, ever write this down without considering the effect this might have on somebody like myself? And it really made me question religion. It really killed me, just killed me. It went to my core; it really wasn't that I took it personally or that I thought my decision was wrong, but it really made me question my basic core. I kept saying to myself, this person is not representative of the whole tribe and he can't be a godly person, because he doesn't understand what it could do to a person whose whole purpose is to bring life and love into a family. It got me confused, and the last thing I needed to be was confused about this.

Lisa was very helpful. She said one of the nicest things about Judaism is all the interpretations; everybody has their own interpretations, and we can take whatever we need. She also said that the person who wrote it didn't talk about what charity, life, giving, sharing, and love are all about. The book went in the garbage. I know AID was the right decision for us.

I think we'll make damn good parents. I feel responsible already. We laughed when Lisa paid the bill for the cat we adopted from the ASPCA. She said, "Now it's *my* cat! I have the canceled check to prove it." And I said, "I have the canceled check to prove that I paid for AID! So it's *my* baby!" The only people who know it isn't are Dr. W. and Vicky, our support group, and my sister and her lover. The child will absolutely be told that it's *my* child. I've never had any other thought about it. Some guy gave a donation—thank you very much. That's where it ends.

In our hearts there was never a donor—it was medicine. And that keeps me strong. I still get inklings once in a while, but I don't feel the failure as much any more. I lost out on the genetic fathering, and I didn't want to lose this experience.

I always thought that what would clear up everything would be the child itself. I'm starting to feel incredibly good about the child. I've shared the child. I've no doubts about who the daddy is—*I'm* the daddy! The kid knows me already.

Lisa: It always moves when Eric comes over to talk to it through my belly. There is no question in my mind—Eric is the father.

I'm just so happy we wound up doing what we did. Very

seldom am I totally happy with the way I've handled a situation. I think we did good. I'm proud of us.

ERIC: When I was a little kid, I always thought I was weird because I used to fantasize about having a wife and a child. When someone pulled the cord on me and put up a roadblock and said, "Stop! You can't do that!" we found alternatives. And taking those choices along the road and getting to where we are now has made me feel this amazing closeness to Lisa. This child that isn't even born yet has brought us a whole lot closer than we ever were. It's really a commitment to a relationship. It's really a commitment to life.

SOCIAL OPTIONS

When a couple has exhausted all the medical or genetic options available to them, the only options that remain are the social options—child-free living or adoption. Again, coming to the point of saying "enough is enough" can be a long, tedious process. But this process does help the couple decide whether they think they can live happily ever after without children.

The most difficult decision for me was the decision to stop. I was on vacation in one of my favorite places thinking things out. I simply decided that I did not want to invest any more of my time, money, and particularly my emotions toward it. If I look at my life realistically, it is complete enough; I do not have to beat my head against a wall to have a child. And I am not sure that a child will enhance my life or make it more difficult.

It must have been brewing for many months. Things had gotten out of control. Basically what I did by the decision was to reestablish control over my life.

Child-Free Living

You may wonder why anyone who has tried so hard to pursue pregnancy would want to remain child free. It's true that most infertile couples wind up with a child by either pregnancy or adoption, but many do choose to remain child free.

Many people, perhaps without even realizing it, are actually longing for a baby rather than a child, but babies very quickly grow up and become children. Said one woman, "I can't get past the thought of having an infant. I can only think that I want this little baby. When the kid gets to be two or three, it's hard to envision it."

Some couples, if they honestly think about it, may find that they are not particularly interested in sharing their lives with a toddler, much less a teenager—especially one who is not genetically related to them. Child-free living would be a very reasonable option for them.

Some couples may have been ambivalent to begin with and then get so caught up in the pursuit of pregnancy that they forget what their original objections were to having children. In their effort to succeed, they may have lost sight of their original ambivalence. When pregnancy no longer appears to be a realistic option, they may come to the realization that they can live happy, fulfilled lives without having children.

Adoption for some infertile couples is simply out of the question. For them, child-free living can be a satisfactory solution. Of course it does help if there are children around that they can enjoy.

My husband had two kids from a previous marriage and didn't want more children when I married him, but I convinced him to try. He turned out to have a varicocele and agreed to have it surgically removed. We then did AIH for six years and nothing happened. I am a DES daughter, and that could also be a cause of our infertility. I finally conceived two years ago on a cycle when we didn't do AIH. It turned out to be an ectopic pregnancy. It took me a long time to get over the pregnancy loss. On the day the baby was supposed to be born, my husband and I decided to go to where my grandfather was buried, and we buried a little pair of booties. I felt that that helped complete the emotion.

So we were down to, "What now?" I decided to be child-free. I'm thirty-eight and since we're not using birth control, if I do become pregnant, that would be great. But when I'm forty, I'll start using birth control.

I don't feel 100 percent good about my decision. I heard a talk at an infertility symposium that no decision is 100 percent—that if it's eighty-twenty, you should feel good about the decision. I feel 80 percent good about my decision.

If my husband would agree to adopt, I would do that. But he is adamant about not adopting. You have to decide what is good for your marriage, and my marriage is more important than pushing this thing of having a child. Perhaps it's because I'm older and live in the city that I don't feel so left out of that world of mothers and children. If I lived in the suburbs, it might be different.

I don't want a child that much now. I went back to school and got a social-work degree, and now I'm a therapist and work with the disabled. My route was to get myself more professionally satisfied and not wallow in trying to have a baby. I'm really happy. I'm not like those who are really sad and can't imagine life without that role. My job is a very nurturing one. And I feel creative—you can be creative in one way when you can't in another.

Also, I'm very integrated into the role of stepmother—my husband's kids are sixteen and nineteen. So I'm a part-time parent and very into my career. Of course, I would like to have a child of my own if I could. But someday I'll be a grandmother, and that will be nice.

I'm much more comfortable now. It's much less painful to be around pregnant women. I don't cry any more. It's not central to my life any more.

Adoption

Many people have a difficult time giving up their pursuit of pregnancy, even in the face of a negative prognosis and constant defeat. They are afraid that if they don't conceive, they will never be parents—that adoption is not really an option for them because they can't get a healthy baby of their own race, or even if they can, it will take too long.

Contrary to popular belief, there are many healthy, newborn babies of *every* race, including caucasian, who are available for adoption. It is true that most adoption agencies have a shortage of newborn white babies, so if that is what you prefer, you have another excellent option, private adoption. More and more couples today are turning to private adoption.

It is true that since legalized abortion, many women who might have given up their babies for adoption in the past are now having abortions. And many others are choosing to keep their babies. Some, however, who may be willing to give up their child for adoption, don't want to deal with the bureaucracy and red tape of the adoption agencies. Through private adoption (also known as independent adoption), which is legal in most states, not only can they choose the couples themselves, through friends, a lawyer, a physician, or even a newspaper ad.

The other fear, that it takes years to adopt a newborn baby, is also not justified. Through either private adoption or another excellent alternative, foreign adoption, the process can and often does take less than a year. One woman told me that after her third miscarriage she came home from the hospital on a Saturday, started making phone calls from her bed to everyone she knew telling them she wanted to adopt a baby, and by Thursday got a call from a lawyer she didn't know (he was the adoption lawyer of the cousin of a friend of a friend). He had heard she was looking for a baby to adopt, and there was a pregnant woman in her eighth month sitting in his office who wanted to give her baby up for adoption. They adopted the baby the next month! Obviously, not all private adoptions happen this quickly, but many do take less time than the nine months most women have to wait to give birth.

We had pretty much been through everything that Western medicine had to offer to help us conceive—we even tried *in vitro* fertilization, and it didn't work. They told me to try again, but I felt like emotionally it was really draining. We came back from it not working and said, "This is absurd, we want to be parents!" Then we just switched gears and went very much toward adoption. We had done a lot of mourning, so all that was pretty much past. Once we turned the tables we were in gear, and it felt wonderful!

We found our child three months from the day we decided to adopt. We put ads in thirteen newspapers and made them very much from our gut, because we realized we were hoping to deal with people on the gut level. And one of us was always home to answer the phone—we didn't use an answering machine. It turned out, however, that the women did prefer to talk to me rather than my husband. We got a number of calls, and finally we got the *right* call. The connection really felt terrific—we even sounded like we looked alike and thought alike. And then he was born. We went through some trauma about that; we were really scared about whether he would really be ours. We were afraid the birth mother would not give him up. But she did, and we picked up our son at the hospital when he was four days old.

Not only was this woman able to adopt very quickly, but with perseverance she was able to overcome another common objection to adoption—that it robs the mother of the chance to enjoy breast-feeding.

I had known from the minute we decided to adopt that I really wanted to try to breast-feed; that intimacy was something I really wanted. So at that point I started to do manual massage in the shower or if I was watching TV. I had a few drops of milk before our baby arrived.

The day we brought him home from the hospital, I started nursing him using Lact-Aid, a device that holds formula in a pouch. The baby then sucks simultaneously the breast and a tube alongside of the nipple, allowing him to get enough formula and breast milk for a feeding. The sucking stimulates the breast to produce more milk.

In the beginning it was difficult, but I knew it was often hard for mothers who give birth to their babies. I did get some help from Lact-Acid and La Leche League. The one thing I was absolutely clear about was that I wasn't going to get hooked into thinking that this was a success or failure by how much milk I got. The important thing to me was the intimacy with him. And it has certainly helped me feel a biological connection to him. He's two and I'm still nursing—with the Lact-Aid. It's an absolutely thrilling thing to do.

Even when told the realities about adoption, some people have great difficulties in accepting the idea of raising a child that is not biologically their own. The decision to adopt is a very personal decision, and some couples can never accept the idea of raising someone else's child. For them, it's probably best not to adopt, especially if both spouses feel so negative. However, difficulties can arise when one spouse is willing to pursue adoption and the other is not.

Facing the possibility of adopting is traumatic for many couples; they are confronted with their failure to "reproduce themselves," and this means giving up their dreams of having their own child with their genes and their looks. And for many, these are hard dreams to relinquish.

Frequently, one spouse feels more positively about adoption and more easily accepts the reality that this is probably the only way they are ever going to have children, whereas the other spouse is opposed to the idea. More often than not, it is the husband who has a harder time accepting the notion of adoption.

This month I brought up the subject of adoption with my husband for the very first time. It was bad news; he was so against that one, he didn't even want to discuss it. He said, "If we can't have our own children, I don't want anybody else's children. And besides, there are no healthy, normal, intellectually curious caucasian babies up for adoption."

If the decision to adopt is not mutually made, it is bound to cause conflict in the marriage. As one woman put it, "My husband is angry at me for ultimately deciding that my way of dealing with the infertility is to render it a nonproblem by adopting."

Adoption can be not only an issue of debate, but one of control as well.

After my laparoscopy, the doctor said there was no hope, and my husband said, "If we're not going to be able to conceive, I don't want to adopt for two years." That's when I felt this thing is the pits. I'm now getting punished—I can't conceive and therefore I can't get to have what I want, a baby.

A spouse's refusal to consider adoption might even prompt someone to consider divorce.

There were times I thought I might leave him because of his

reluctance to look into adoption. I really considered leaving and finding a man who was divorced with two kids, because Tim is just not that anxious to have a family.

What can be done if a couple disagrees about adoption—or any of the other options, for that matter? The couple could certainly benefit from some sort of counseling at that point, from either a marriage or an infertility counselor.

My wife came to the idea of adopting much sooner than I did. When she first brought it up, I didn't want to talk about it or I was grumpy and said it was awful and threw out all the possible objections to it. I knew at the back of my mind there was no question about the fact that we both wanted kids. So I knew I was going to come around eventually, but I had to be dragged kicking and screaming, and I ended up talking to an infertility counselor. It was a big struggle, but we finally agreed to adopt. And now we're happy with both that decision *and* our adopted daughter.

According to psychotherapist Dr. Kate Gorman:

It's legitimate for one spouse to say, "I need more time to decide about this." But that doesn't mean the other spouse should have to continue pursuing treatments unless she or he is physically and emotionally able to do so.

One of the best ways to help someone decide about adopting is to gather information—to go together to meetings on adoption where people who have adopted or dealt with adoption talk about it in a very nonthreatening way. In that way they can begin to filter out which objections they have to adoption are valid and which are not. For example, someone might say, "We're never going to stop pursuing treatment, because adoption takes ten years." When they learn that adoption of a healthy newborn can take less than a year, they may have a more positive attitude.

Talking to other people who have adopted, or are planning to do so, can often help someone decide that adoption is not such a bad idea after all.

My wife and I have friends who are getting a four-month-old baby from India next month. The wife is very excited about it and actually said that if she were told she could have a baby of her own and had a choice between the two, she would want to follow through with the adoption. It made me feel that there's no reason why that experience can't be as enriching as having your own child. That kind of opened my mind to adoption.

I'm trying to keep a positive attitude. If that means shifting from feeling we could have our own child to an alternative—having a child another way—I'll try to make that shift and pull it off in a way that is not going to make us have a lot of bad feelings. That issue is to have a kid; I don't want to get bogged down feeling lousy about it.

Realizing that adoption does not necessarily rule out the possibility of pursuing pregnancy again at some later date helps some couples accept the adoption options.

I was thinking about adoption much more than Ted was, mainly because I wanted out. I felt like I was in a cage. At first his attitude was, "Yes, maybe if we can't have a child we will adopt." But only if there was absolutely no hope of conceiving —admitting you're going to adopt was the ultimate failure.

And then about six months later, adoption shifted to something one could possibly do and still try to get pregnant—it didn't rule out having a biological child. And then ultimately when I decided it wasn't worth trying to conceive any more, it became the only option.

However, if you go into adoption with the idea that it will help you get pregnant, you're not only deluding yourself but setting yourself up for disappointment, since most women who adopt never do become pregnant (see chapter 6).

When the decision is finally made to adopt, it is often followed by a sense of relief. As one woman put it, "I really feel that a big weight has been taken off my shoulders. It's like coming out of the closet. I don't think I've felt so good about myself in years."

Once the decision is made to adopt, infertility can begin to fade into the background and lose its hold on the couple's life. The couple may also discover that just the prospect of a future adoption can be exhilarating.

I must say, I really feel better at this point having stopped, because we really feel we've done what we could do, and that's the best anyone can do. . . . Just this last week or so, I began to have hope for the future. I don't know what day of the month it is. I'm forgetting the names of the medicines. I'm really saying I don't want to be thinking about this any more. I used to know everything so well. But I'm sure that's because we're so close to adoption—it's like something else to put our minds to.

I'm collecting little baby clothes. I feel like I'm playing house, but I'm thrilled. I've been collecting cradles and rockers and little baths and I've been knitting little baby things, and we don't even know when the baby is going to arrive. It could be next month, it could be the summer, it could be the fall. But now I feel legitimate and reasonable to make plans, because we are going to have a baby!

Most people who actively pursue pregnancy do so, at least in part, because they think they will make good parents; they feel they have a lot to offer a child. Not only does adoption provide couples with the opportunity to do just that—be good parents—it allows them to provide a loving home for a child who may otherwise not have one. Regardless of the reasons a child is put up for adoption, it cannot be cared for by its biological parents and needs to be adopted into another family in order to have a normal life.

THE COOPERS

Neither the surgery nor the danazol treatment for Mai Li's endometriosis had worked so far to get her pregnant. She and Roy made an appointment with Dr. S. to discuss what they should do next—pursue more medical treatment, or pursue adoption.

ROY: When we went to see Dr. S., he was very emphatic and pulled no punches. Wishy-washy attitudes are not part of his repertoire. He started out by saying, "Things do not look good; I'm not happy with what I see, I'm not happy with what has happened. Now where do we go from here?" He then suggested a second-look laparoscopy.

I was really upset and discouraged. That evening we went out to eat, and I started having fantasies about getting drunk and destroying the restaurant. I was furious and kept thinking, It's unfair, it's so goddamn unfair!

That night I had a dream. It was in three parts. In the first part my male cat brought home a puppy to play with. My cat is gray and white, and the puppy was golden. The cat licked it a lot. In the second part of the dream, Mai Li and I were walking down a country road. We were holding each other with a tenderness and supportiveness and closeness that accompanies grief and sadness. In the last part my mother had just died, and I was required to put little pieces of black tape onto a purple cloth attached to the coffin. I felt the dream represented the death of biological motherhood, but opened us up for the possibility of adoption. When I woke up the next morning, I knew it was time to seriously pursue this option.

MAI LI: From the time we found out that I had blocked tubes, we had always thought of adoption as our safety net. But when it came time to actually do something about it, we vacillated a lot. But finally we came to the point where we wanted to do it more than we didn't. Also, since there seemed to be nothing more we could do medically, we thought at least we would be doing something positive.

At RESOLVE, we had been hearing a lot about private adoption; quite a few of the members had successfully adopted newborn white babies. But since we *preferred* a racially mixed child—Asian-causcasian—we thought we would be better off with an adoption agency. So once again I hit the Yellow Pages. I was really gung-ho! Adoption agencies, oh, boy! I felt energized and good and productive about it.

ROY: I felt anxious. As positive a move as it was, it was an anxiety-provoking situation.

MAI LI: The next day I thought, Oh, I really don't want to do this. I want to get pregnant! I don't want to adopt. And I felt that way for a while, but then realized that since it would probably take several years to adopt a baby, I still had a chance to get pregnant. So we started calling up agencies.

ROY: The first one we called told us on the phone that we

were too old, even though Mai Li was only thirty-one. I guess they thought a forty-one-year-old man was too old to be a father! We were finally able to get an interview at the second agency we called.

I was very nervous going there. When we arrived, we were called into this woman's office. She was very striking and had on this beautiful jewelry—like Aztec Indian jewelry. It made a positive impression on me, that here was a woman of culture and taste.

She started asking us questions about our backgrounds and routine questions about age, height, weight, religion, medical problems, and so on. Then she said to us, "Describe your relationship—what's good about your relationship, what's bad about your relationship. Tell me all the things you like about each other and all the things you don't like about each other." I can't tell you how upsetting it was.

We were then exposed to a barrage of questions about the potential child. Would we accept a child who was the product of incest? Would we accept a child who was the product of rape? Would we accept a child whose mother was on heroin? On and on and on.

I felt we were victims of necessity—we needed to be there. We wanted desperately to be accepted by this agency. It wasn't like we had another agency lined up. One agency had already turned us down because we were too old. We were both very anxious. What if this door is closed, the safety net taken away? And all the time I kept thinking, I *don't* want a product of incest. I *don't* want the child of a heroin addict.

We finally said no to all those questions. But I was very apprehensive about whether our saying no would eliminate the possibility of getting a child from them. So I finally said to her, "I don't know what you want, but I was brought up in a household with a mentally retarded sister, and it was a very painful experience to me. The idea of repeating it is just too painful." I couldn't do what my parents did. I just couldn't do it.

MAI LI: When we left, she said she would get back to us. She said the committee would review our case and we would receive a letter in about two weeks. We both turned out not to like the woman at all—she turned out to be very cold. She had introduced herself to us by her first and last names and after two hours of interviewing, Roy asked if he could call her by her first name. She said, "No!"—she was that kind of person. The whole experience was disgusting. When we left all we could talk about was how we didn't like that woman.

Two weeks later we got a letter that said, "After careful consideration, the committee has decided that it would be too difficult and take too long to find a child for you, so we cannot accept you on our list." I had expected that rejection.

ROY: We were both really upset, but then a lawyer friend helped us get an interview at another agency.

MAI LI: That interview process was totally different. Instead of one two-hour interview, it was a series of interviews. The initial interview was just a get-acquainted introduction-to-the-process interview to see if we wanted to go through with the application. This adoption supervisor wasn't as well dressed as the first one, but she was much nicer! We called her by her first name, Claire, and she was very warm and pleasant. The questions were similar and we answered the same way, but it was a very different experience—much more pleasant.

Then she scheduled a couple's interview, a private interview with Roy, one with me, and a home visit over the next couple of months. We also had to have physical exams.

ROY: We were very uptight about the home study. Mai Li was especially concerned, because we had a very nontraditional life-style; we lived in a loft with video equipment all over the place.

MAI LI: Claire told us that the home studies had changed since the fifties, and most people didn't realize that. They used to look for the traditional family—and no dirt under the sofa. But now they look for a home where the child would be brought up in a nurturing, loving way.

ROY: Even though we did feel that our life-style was a bit unconventional, I basically felt it was a very positive life-style. Mai Li would say things like, "Who lives in a loft? She'll think we're crazy!" I would say, "But this is a child's paradise! It'll have room to run around and not be confined."

MAI LI: I felt reasonably confident that Roy and I would

make good parents and that anybody with any intelligence could see that.

ROY: Before she came, we did clean and straighten up a lot. We served her lunch, and the visit went smoothly and quickly. She told us that the committee would make their decision within thirty days.

MAI LI: By then I was president of RESOLVE. We were putting together a meeting on adoption, so I called up Claire and asked her to be on the panel. She was very eager to do that, and it went very well.

A few weeks later we got a letter from her saying we were placed on her waiting list. That was a real coincidence, but somehow I kept thinking, the more aggressive you are in life, the more things happen for you.

We were told that once they accepted you they were committed to placing a child with you. They said that they placed five kids a year, and the average time waiting for a baby was three to five years.

ROY: And they told us up front that it was not like the bakery where they gave you a number and it's first come, first served, but that they tried to place the *right* child in the *right* family.

MAI LI: Once we were accepted, we breathed a sigh of relief. We now had all bases covered. We knew someday we would be parents. If nothing panned out with a pregnancy, we would be able to adopt within five years. In the meantime, we could keep working on our infertility.

Dr. S. had nothing more to suggest except another laparoscopy, so Roy and Mai Li made an appointment to have a consultation with another doctor, Dr. E. They had heard a lot of good things about him at RESOLVE—that he was a highly qualified reproductive endocrinologist and also was very nice and personable, a real bonus. And several of the RESOLVE members who had used him had gotten pregnant.

MAI LI: A friend of ours who went to Dr. E. said that he could even get the operating table pregnant!

ROY: I had some ambivalence about seeing Dr. E., the miracle worker. I was skeptical. I thought that if Dr. S. felt he couldn't do anything, what could Dr. E. possibly do?

MAI LI: When we went to see Dr. E., he was as nice and knowledgeable as everyone said. He was fairly optimistic, and I felt optimistic again because I was seeing a new doctor who had new ideas and approaches. He had a lot of things he wanted to try. He did another hysterosalpingogram and an endometrial biopsy, which I had never had, and sent me for a sonogram, and did some postcoital exams—one procedure a month. He then decided to try me on a fertility drug, Clomid. I was very excited when he suggested Clomid; it was another thing to try. The most upsetting thing for me was to have nothing left to try. As long as you have something to try, there's hope.

The adoption process was taking as long as the infertility workup, so we had them running neck and neck. It was like a race—which process would win or come out more favorably. Something had to happen one way or the other.

After I had been on Clomid for two months with no pregnancy, I started to get discouraged again. I hadn't heard from Claire in about six months, so I called her up to see if there was any progress on our case.

I told her we were really still interested in a child; basically it was a cover-up for saying, "Please don't forget about me. I'm still here and I still want a child." We talked for a long time and after a while she said, "By the way, you mentioned that you wanted an oriental-caucasian mixture." I said that was right. She said, "Does that mean any oriental?" And I said, "Well, I guess so," and I started to reel off a list of all the orientals I could think of and I said, "Chinese, yes; Japanese, yes; Vietnamese, yes." And she interrupted and said, "Well, what about something like Indonesian?" I got excited—she was too specific about the race, so I knew instantly that she had something specific in mind for us. I told her, "I think that would be wonderful, but I have to check with Roy and I'll get back to you." I called Roy and said, "I spoke to Claire and she has a child in mind for us who will be half Indonesian."

ROY: I said, "Indonesian . . . I don't think I've ever even *met* an Indonesian."

Then I had this phenomenal experience. I got on a bus a few days later, and a woman with a beautiful little girl also got on. The woman had her hands full of packages and the kid needed help getting up on the seat, so I helped her up. And I turned to the mother and said, "This kid is the most exquisite child I have ever seen in my entire life!" I couldn't believe how gorgeous this kid was. Then I said to the mother, "What nationality is this child?" And the mother said, "We're Indonesian." Then I started talking to her about the Indonesian people. I couldn't wait to get to my stop. When I got off the bus I ran to the house and up the steps and said, "Mai Li, Mai Li, call them up, tell them an Indonesian would be great!!"

MAI LI: I called Claire back and said, "Roy and I talked about this, and we've decided that an Indonesian-caucasian child would be very welcome in our home." And she said, "Well, that's nice. You'll be hearing from us."

I suspected that there was a pregnant woman Claire was counseling and that we had quite a bit of time yet before anything happened. While I was happy that there would be a baby that was potentially available to us, I didn't want to get too excited, because pregnant women are known to change their minds. We would also have plenty of time to change *our* minds if I got pregnant or if we chickened out—even if the woman gave birth in a few months, the baby would have to be in a foster home for about six months until it could legally be placed with adoptive parents.

Roy and I discussed whether we could love a child that was not biologically ours. We didn't know to determine that, so I devised these little experiments. I would go around and meet or see babies and I would fantasize that I would take them home. And after doing that enough times, I came to the conclusion that I could love *any* child. So that made me feel better about adopting and about my capacity to love that child.

ROY: I was always comfortable about the idea of adopting. In the fifties when abortion was illegal, all my friends talked about having one kid and adopting another. That was years behind me, and I hadn't thought about it for a while. But I had been around kids a lot and loved kids.

MAI LI: I continued to take Clomid. We were still hoping I might get pregnant.

A few months after I had spoken to Claire, we were about to leave for a weekend in the country and the phone rang. Roy answered it. It was Claire. Roy said, "Mai Li, you'd better pick up the other phone." So I picked up the other phone and said, "Hi, how are you?" and she said, "How are *you*?" I said, "Fine," and she said, "Well, you're going to feel a lot better." And I said, "Really?" And she said, "We have a little girl we'd like you to consider." And I said, "What kind of little girl? Tell me about her." And she said, "She's half Indonesian and half caucasian. She's four months old, and she's in foster care."

My first reaction was, I'm not ready for this decision. I asked when this event would happen if we decided to take the child. And she said, "You can take the child home next week." That really got us reeling! Six months' preparation is one thing, but one week! She said, "Let's make an appointment and talk about it." So we made an appointment to see her on the following Wednesday.

ROY: I was in shock. And the phone call came at a time when there were a lot of important financial and career decisions we had to make in our lives. I felt *very* pressured.

MAI LI: When we got to the country, we took a walk and sat at the edge of a pond and talked. It was a *monumental* decision. We were going to have to pick up the phone and make a call that was going to change the rest of our lives! What if we passed on this child? We might never have another opportunity like this again. I felt that God was giving us this child —she was exactly what we wanted. It was too perfect, and I was afraid of missing the opportunity. I wanted a child. I wanted to adopt her, but I also had reservations and was very ambivalent.

We had a huge fight in the car on the way home from the country. My sense was that Roy was leaning toward refusing the adoption, which frightened me, and I started to want it more. I kind of suppressed my ambivalences to try to convince him that we *must* have this child. I thought my infertility was absolute; Roy didn't.

ROY: I got really angry because I thought that the very act of adopting was going to put a stop to our attempting to have our own biological child. That this was the end. That we had no chance. I wasn't sure I was there yet. I wasn't prepared.

And I felt like I had been an asshole all this time. It's like you're going out with some girl and you really love her and really care for her and all of a sudden she says, "Get lost, I always thought you were a shmuck!" That's the way I felt. I had all this hope in what we were doing. There was a lot invested—the trips to the doctor, the surgery, the drugs—all this and it came to nothing.

If Mai Li had come to me and said, "Roy, you've got to understand, we've been trying this for three years now and it's not hopeful—I've just reached the point where I can't take it any more. I'm wiped out," I wouldn't have been so upset. But the *way* she expressed it—she said, "What are you, crazy? We've been doing this for three and a half years—it's not going to happen! Sooner the moon will be blue than I'll get pregnant!"—that just left me feeling that I was this clown being dragged along for the ride. It made me crazy! So it didn't have to do with the issue of whether to adopt. It stirred up other passions in me.

MAI LI: The whole underlying thing was, we were tremendously anxious and our nerves were raw. We were emotionally crazed. We finally worked out a compromise. I would have a pregnancy test, since I had taken Clomid that month and hadn't gotten my period yet. If it came back negative, we would go ahead with this adoption. I had the test on Monday. It came back negative.

We met with Claire on Wednesday, and she showed us pictures of the child. We both thought she was really homely. I said to Claire, "Oh, she's sweet." It was a lie. She said we could come on Monday and pick up the child. We said, "Fine." I didn't want her to know we were ambivalent.

ROY: But we knew deep down that we wanted this child. Underneath it all, we wanted to be parents. We really wanted *this* child. All the background stuff sounded good—the mother was educated, was from a middle-class family, and had had good prenatal care.

MAI LI: And I was pleased that she was only four months old. The agency said the average age for adoption was six months old. But I was still uncertain as to whether we had made the right decision. I called friends of ours from RE-SOLVE who had adopted a few months earlier and I said, "I don't know if I want to take this child." The husband, who is a lawyer, said that they had felt the same way and that you're not legally obligated to keep the child until you formally adopt, and that can take six months to a year. I called other friends who had adopted and asked lots of questions and said things like, "What if this child is ugly? We saw the pictures; she's not so pretty." One friend said her adopted daughter from Korea had looked deformed in the pictures, and she had even showed the pictures to a pediatrician. Her daughter turned out to be gorgeous. She also said, "Your child will be well-dressed, have a great haircut—she's going to look wonderful!" So that was reassuring. We were looking for support for this decision we really hadn't made yet.

ROY: I called my mother and said we were adopting this baby and she was homely. It didn't faze my mother at all. She said, "Listen, don't worry about that, take the baby. This is *so* important. Stop already. I feel so bad for you and all you've been up against. You'll take this baby and you'll have a *child*, a family." She was very supportive—it was really wonderful.

MAI LI: Between Wednesday and Friday night, we slowly came to the decision we were going to do it. Over the weekend, we cleaned out my work room and painted it, put up curtains, bought a crib and a changing table. I was vacillating between being terribly excited and terribly frightened and numb in between.

ROY: The more work we put into getting ready for the baby, the more excited we became.

MAI LI: I called a friend who had had a baby nine months before and said, "We're going to adopt a baby and pick her up on Monday!" And she said, "Oh, that's wonderful! Do you need some things?" I said yes, and she started giving me a layette list and then said, "Don't buy stretchies, a playpen, or an infant seat; I'll bring you mine." On Saturday morning she and her husband came up with a car full of baby things. That was very moving, very touching. People really rallied round us and were very supportive and wonderful.

The joy and the tears and the support made it much easier—we were caught up in all that enthusiasm in spite of our fears. When we walked out of our loft Monday morning to get her, I literally walked into the wall!

ROY: By the time we walked into that office to get the baby, I was never so excited in my life! Excitement and anxiety. It was an incredibly intense emotional experience. I was on the verge of running, crying, grabbing on to something, going forward, running away from it.

MAI LI: We were so excited! It was like opening night. I had this kind of heady, giddy feeling of waiting for the curtains to open—that I was in the play but I didn't know what I was going to say. We sat down and Claire gave us some more information and finally said, "Well, should I get her?" We said, "Sure!"

ROY: I almost passed out from excitement! It was very thrilling. But I was also prepared for some disappointment based on those photos. I was also afraid they were going to give me this child that I wasn't going to love so much. Somehow it was the final hand in the game of infertility—it was the last card. OK, draw from the adoptive pile and you get ugly baby. It was adding insult to injury.

We were sitting there in that room, and the foster mother brought in this child that was absolutely *gorgeous*! She was so beautiful! I just couldn't believe it. I just kept looking at her and thinking, Oh, my God! This is *our baby*! I melted.

MAI LI: She was like a vision. She was smiling, beautiful, and alert, and she wasn't crying or clinging. She couldn't have been more wonderful! I started to cry. Everyone in the room was crying!

Claire handed her to me, and Roy took pictures. I felt immediately protective. I was overwhelmed with all kinds of emotions!

ROY: We took a cab home and I told the cab driver, "Please drive very carefully because we have a *very special* child in here."

MAI LI: She fell asleep in the cab, so when we got home we

put her in her new crib. We named our daughter Lili—a name in both cultures.

ROY: I can't imagine loving a child more than we love Lili, and I can't imagine any child in the world being more loved.

MAI LI: And I can't imagine that Roy and I could have produced a more wonderful child than Lili. I don't think biologically we could have done as well—we really lucked out! I'm in love. It's a romance—a brand-new romance in my life.

ROY: I walk around feeling blessed. I have a feeling that if there is a God, he was kind of watching out up there and he said, "Make these people infertile, because they deserve a special child and I have a special kid in reserve for them." And that special kid is our daughter, Lili.

APPENDIX A

GLOSSARY

Adhesions: Scar tissues that attach to the surfaces of organs.

AID: Artificial insemination with donor sperm. The process of placing the sperm from a man other than the husband in a woman's vagina or cervix with the use of medical instruments.

AIDS: Acquired immune deficiency syndrome. A disorder of the immune system not to be confused with AID (artificial insemination with donor sperm).

AIH: Artificial insemination with husband's sperm. The process of placing the husband's sperm into the woman's vagina or cervix with the use of medical instruments.

Amniocentesis: A medical procedure in which a small amount of amniotic fluid is removed by needle from the uterus of a pregnant woman. The fluid is then analyzed to detect genetic abnormalities in the growing fetus.

Androgens: Male sex hormones.

Andrologist: A physician who specializes in the study of male sex hormones.

Anovulation: The absence of ovulation.

Artificial insemination: The introduction of sperm from husband (AIH) or donor (AID) into the vagina or cervix of a woman by means of medical instruments.

Aspermia: The absence of sperm in the semen. Also called azoospermia.

Azoospermia: The absence of sperm in the semen.

Basal body temperature (BBT): A temperature taken orally or rectally the first thing in the morning, before any activity. When the BBT is taken daily by a woman, it charts her menstrual cycle and gives some indication of ovulation and presence of certain hormones.

Cervix: The neck or opening of the uterus.

Cervical mucus: Secretions produced by the cervix that vary in viscosity according to the phase of the menstrual cycle.

Clomid: The brand name for clomiphene citrate, a synthetic drug commonly used to treat infertility because it stimulates ovulation.

Culdoscopy: A surgical procedure in which a telescope-like instrument is inserted through a small incision in the vagina. The ovaries, fallopian tubes, and uterus can then be directly visualized. This procedure, while less popular than a laparoscopy, is used to diagnose and sometimes correct structural causes of infertility.

Danazol (Danocrine): A drug commonly used to treat endometriosis by temporarily suppressing ovulation. Danazol is the generic name; Danocrine a brand name.

Donor insemination: See AID (artificial insemination with donor sperm).

Ectopic pregnancy: A pregnancy that implants outside the uterus. This is a potentially life-threatening situation that always requires immediate medical attention and often surgery.

Ejaculation: The ejection of semen and sperm from the penis during orgasm.

Embryo: The developing human organism from one week after conception to the end of the second month, when it becomes a fetus.

Endocrine system: A system of glands in the body that produce hormones. The endocrine system includes the ovaries, testes, pituitary, parathyroid, thyroid, and adrenal glands.

Endocrinologist: A physician specializing in the treatment of diseases of the hormonal (endocrine) system.

Endometriosis: A disease in which pieces of the uterine lining (endometrium) grow outside the uterus in such places as the fallopian tubes, ovaries, or abdominal cavity. This condition can cause pain and infertility.

Endometrial biopsy: A diagnostic office procedure in which a small sample of the lining of the uterus (endometrium) is removed and then examined under a microscope for evidence of the presence or absence of certain hormones. This helps determine whether a woman ovulates or has hormonal imbalances.

Endoscopy: A surgical procedure in which a telescopelike instrument is inserted through the abdomon (laparoscopy) or vagina (culdoscopy) to visualize the ovaries, uterus, and fallopian tubes. This procedure is used to diagnose and sometimes correct the structural causes of infertility.

Estrogen: The primary female hormone, produced mainly in the ovaries after puberty until menopause.

Estradiol: The major circulation estrogen hormone produced in the ovary and necessary for ovulation.

Fallopian tubes: A pair of narrow tubes that pick up the egg from the ovary and carry it to the uterus for implantation. The egg is normally fertilized in a fallopian tube before it travels to the uterus.

Fertilization: The penetration of an egg by a sperm.

Fetus: The developing human organism after the embryo stage, from the end of the second month until birth.

Fibroid tumor: A benign (noncancerous) tumor that grows in the uterine wall. Also called a myoma.

Fibroids: See Fibroid tumor.

Follicle: Egg sac in the ovary that contains the immature egg (oocyte).

FSH (follicle stimulating hormone): A hormone produced by the pituitary gland that stimulates the production of sperm in males and eggs in females.

Gamete: A reproductive cell in either the male (sperm) or female (egg).

Genetic: Determined by heredity.

Gonadotropin: Pituitary hormones (FSH and LH) that stimulate the production of sperm in males and eggs in females.

Gynecologist: A physician who specializes in diagnosis and treatment of diseases of the female reproductive system.

Hamster egg penetration test: The penetration ability of a human sperm egg is tested by having it attempt to penetrate a hamster egg.

HCG (human chorionic gonadotropin): A hormone secreted by the placenta during pregnancy. HCG is often given by injection after Clomid or Pergonal in order to trigger ovulation. It is also the hormone measured in pregnancy tests that determines whether a woman is pregnant.

HMG (human menopausal gonadotropin): The generic name for the fertility drug, Pergonal. HMG, which contains FSH and LH, is extracted from the urine of postmenopausal women and is given by injection to women to stimulate egg production. It has also been used experimentally in men to stimulate sperm production.

Hormone: A chemical produced by an endocrine gland.

Husband insemination: See AIH (artificial insemination with husband's sperm).

Hysterosalpingogram: A diagnostic x-ray procedure in which radiopaque dye is injected through the cervix into the uterus and fallopian tubes to determine whether the tubes are open (patent) and the uterus is normally shaped.

Implantation: The embedding of the fertilized egg into the lining of the uterus.

Impotence: The inability of the male to have or maintain an erection.

Infertility: The inability to conceive or maintain a pregnancy after one year of regular unprotected intercourse.

Intrauterine insemination: Artificial insemination in which the sperm is inserted through the cervix into the uterus rather than into the vagina. This technique should only be done with the washed sperm. See Sperm washing.

In vitro: Outside the body, usually in a glass test tube or Petri dish.

In vitro **fertilization (IVF):** A woman's eggs are surgically removed from her ovaries and are placed in a Petri dish with her husband's (or a donor's) sperm. If the egg becomes fertilized and divides into eight cells, it is then transferred into the woman's uterus, where it is hoped it will implant and grow into a viable fetus. The babies that result from IVF are often (incorrectly) labeled "test tube babies."

In vivo: In the body.

IUD (intrauterine device): A birth control device that is inserted into a woman's uterus. Thought to be a contributing factor to infertility in some women.

IVF: see *In vitro* fertilization.

Laparoscopy: A surgical procedure in which a telescopelike instrument is inserted through a small incision in the navel to directly visualize the ovaries, fallopian tubes and uterus. This procedure is used to diagnose and sometimes correct structural causes of infertility.

LH (lutenizing hormone): A hormone secreted by the pituitary gland. In women, it causes the mature egg to be released from the ovary (ovulation). In men, it stimulates testosterone production and is necessary for the production of sperm.

Luteal phase: The second phase of the menstrual cycle, after ovulation. Progesterone is produced during the luteal phase, which normally lasts fourteen days, until the onset of menstruation.

Microsurgery: Surgery that is performed with the aid of a microscope and very fine sutures.

Miscarriage: The uninduced loss of a pregnancy before the fetus is viable outside the uterus. Also called spontaneous abortion.

Morphology: The shape and structure of sperm.

Motility: The ability of sperm to move forward.

Obstetrician: A physician who specializes in pregnancy and childbirth.

Oligospermia: Scarcity of sperm in the semen.

Ova: Eggs. The plural of ovum.

Ovary: The female sex gland that is responsible for producing eggs and the female hormones estrogen and progesterone. There are two ovaries, one on either side of the uterus.

Ovulation: The release of the mature egg (ovum) from a follicle in the ovary. This normally occurs in the middle of the menstrual cycle.

Ovum: An egg.

Petri dish: A small glass laboratory dish used, among other purposes, for *in vitro* fertilization.

Pelvic inflammatory disease (PID): An inflammatory disease of the reproductive tract usually caused by an infection.

Pergonal: The brand name of the injectible form of human menopausal gonadotropin (HMG). It is a potent fertility drug that is commonly used to stimulate egg production in females and, experimentally, to increase sperm production in males.

Postcoital test (Sims-Huhner test): A diagnosic test done at midcycle in which a sample of vaginal and cervical secretions or mucus is taken several hours after intercourse. The sample is then looked at under a microscope to determine how many sperm exist and how well they survive in the cervical mucus. The test also gives some indication of the presence and quality of ovulation.

Premature ejaculation: The discharge of sperm from the penis immediately before or just after it enters the vagina.

Progesterone: A female sex hormone produced by the ovaries during the second phase (luteal phase) of the menstrual cycle, after ovulation. It prepares the lining of the uterus for implantation of a fertilized egg. During pregnancy, it is produced by the placenta.

Rubin test: See Tubal insufflation test.

Scrotum: The external sac that contains the testicles.

Secondary infertility: The inability to conceive or carry a pregnancy to term after having previously had at least one successful pregnancy.

Semen: The liquid seminal secretions and sperm that are released from the penis during ejaculation.

Semen analysis: The evaluation of fresh ejaculate under the microscope. This test primarily determines the number of sperm, their ability to move forward (motility), and whether or not they are normally shaped (morphology).

Seminal fluid: See Semen.

Sims-Huhner test: See Postcoital test.

Sonogram: The use of high-frequency sound waves to examine the uterus and ovaries. It is often used to evaluate follicle development prior to ovulation. It can also be used to determine the location and viability of a fetus.

Sperm: Male reproductive cells that are produced in the testicles. Also called spermatozoa.

Sperm antibodies: A substance within the body that kills sperm. Men can have antibodies to their own sperm, and women can have antibodies in their cervical mucus to their husband's sperm.

Sperm washing: A process by which the sperm are separated from the seminal fluid. This technique helps separate good-quality sperm from poor-quality sperm, so it is often used for artificial insemination, especially intrauterine inseminations.

Spontaneous abortion: See Miscarriage.

Sterility: The absolute inability to reproduce. Not to be confused with infertility.

Subfertility: Less than normal fertility. Sometimes used synonymously with infertility.

Surrogate mother: A woman who is contracted to become pregnant by the husband of an infertile woman, to carry the child to term, and after birth to relinquish it for adoption by the infertile couple.

Temperature charts: See Basal body temperature (BBT).

Testes: The male sex glands inside the scrotum that produce sperm and testosterone. Also called testicles.

Testosterone: A male sex hormone produced by the testes.

Testicles: See Testes.

Test tube baby: A baby conceived by *in vitro* fertilization.

Tubal pregnancy: See Ectopic pregnancy.

Tubal insufflation test (Rubin test): A diagnostic test in which a gas (carbon dioxide) is blown into the uterus to determine whether the fallopian tubes are open (patent). This test is less accurate than the hysterosalpingogram, and for the most part has been replaced by it.

Ultrasound: High-frequency sound waves. See Sonogram.

Urologist: A physician who diagnoses and treats diseases of the male reproductive system. They also diagnose and treat diseases of the urinary tract in both males and females.

Uterine insemination: See Intrauterine insemination.

Uterus: The female reproductive organ that houses, protects, and nourishes the growing fetus during pregnancy. Also called womb.

Varicocele: A varicose (enlarged) vein in the testicle that sometimes causes infertility in men.

Varicocelectomy: A surgical procedure used to remove a varicocele.

Vasectomy: A surgical procedure in which a man is rendered permanently sterile by cutting the duct (vas deferens) that runs from the testes into the penis.

Womb: See Uterus.

APPENDIX B

BIBLOGRAPHY

MEDICAL TEXTS ON INFERTILITY
(available in medical bookstores and libraries)

AMELAR, RICHARD D., M.D., DUBIN, LAWRENCE, M.D. and WALSH, PATRICK C. *Male Infertility*. Philadelphia: W.B. Saunders Co., 1977.

BEHRMAN, S.J., M.D. and KISTNER, ROBERT W., M.D. *Progress in Infertility*. Boston: Little, Brown & Co., 1975.

GARCIA, CELSO-RAMON, M.D., MASTROIANNI, LUIGI, M.D., AMELAR, RICHARD, M.D. and DUBIN, LAWRENCE, M.D., eds. *Current Therapy of Infertility, 1984–1985*. Philadelphia: B.C. Decker, Inc., 1984.

JONES, H., M.D., JONES, G.S., M.D., HODGEN, G., M.D. and ROSENWAKS, Z., M.D., eds. *In Vitro Fertilization: Norfolk*. Baltimore: Williams & Wilkins, 1986.

SPEROFF, LEON, M.D., GLASS, ROBERT H., M.D., and KASE, NATHAN G., M.D. *Clinical Gynecologic Endocrinology and Infertility*. Baltimore: W.B. Saunders Co., 1978.

WALLACH, EDWARD E., M.D. and KEMPERS, ROGER D., M.D., *Modern Trends in Infertility and Conception Control*. New York: Harper & Row, 1982.

GENERAL BOOKS ON INFERTILITY

ANDREWS, LORI B., J.D. *New Conceptions.* New York: St. Martins Press, 1984. (Ballantine paperback, 1985)

BARKER, GRAHAM, M.D. *Your Search for Fertility.* William Morrow & Co., 1980.

BELLINA, JOSEPH and WILSON, JOSLEEN. *You Can Have a Baby.* New York: Crown Pub., Inc., 1985.

BLAIS, MADELINE. *They Say You Can't Have a Baby.* New York: W.W. Norton, 1979.

CORSON, ALBERT, L., M.D. *Conquering Infertility.* Norwalk, Conn.: Appleton-Century-Crofts, 1983.

DECKER, ALBERT, M.D. and LOEBL, SUZANNE. *Why Can't We Have a Baby?* New York: Warner Books, 1978.

FULLER, ELIZABETH. *Having Your First Baby After Thirty: A Personal Journey from Infertility to Childbirth.* New York: Dodd Mead & Co., 1983.

GLASS, ROBERT H., M.D. and ERICSSON, RONALD J., PH.D. *Getting Pregnant in the 80's.* U. of California, 1982.

GOLDSTEIN, MARC, M.D. and GELDBERG, MICHAEL, PH.D. *The Vasectomy Book.* Boston: Houghton Mifflin, 1982.

HARRISON, MARY. *Infertility: A Guide for Couples.* Boston: Houghton Mifflin, 1979.

HOWARD, JAMES T., M.D. and SCHULTZ, DODI. *We Want to Have a Baby.* New York: E.P. Dutton, 1979.

LIFCHEZ, AARON S., M.D. and FENTON, JUDITH A. *The Fertility Handbook.* New York: Clarkson N. Potter Inc., 1980.

MAZOR, MIRIAM D., M.D. and SIMONS, HARRIET F., eds. *Infertility: Medical, Emotional and Social Considerations.* New York: Human Sciences Press, 1984.

MENNING, BARBARA ECK. *Infertility: A Guide for the Childless Couple.* Englewood Cliffs, N.J.: Prentice-Hall, 1977.

MITCHARD, JACQUELYN. *Mother Less Child.* New York: W.W. Norton & Co., 1985.

NOFZIGER, MARGARET. *The Fertility Question.* Summerton, Tenn.: The Book Publishing Question, 1982.

OLDER, JULIA. *Endometriosis.* New York: Charles Scribner's, 1984.

PERLOE, MARK, M.D. and CHRISTIE, LINDA GAIL. *Miracle Babies and Other Happy Endings for Couples with Fertility Problems.* New York: Rawson Assoc., 1986.

SALZER, LINDA. *Infertility: How Couples Can Cope.* Boston: G.K. Hall, 1986.

SILBER, SHERMAN, M.D. *How to Get Pregnant.* New York: Warner Books, 1981.

STANGEL, JOHN J., M.D. *Fertility and Conception.* New York: New American Library, 1979.

STIGGER, JUDITH A. *Coping with Infertility*. Minneapolis: Augsburg Publishing House, 1983.

TILTON, NAN, TILTON, TODD and MOORE, GAYLEN. *Making Miracles: In Vitro Fertilization*. New York: Doubleday, 1985.

WHITE, KAROL. *What to Do When You Think You Can't Have a Baby*. Garden City, N.Y.: Doubleday, 1981.

BOOKS ON MISCARRIAGES AND PREGNANCY LOSS

BERG, BARBARA. *Nothing to Cry About*. New York: Seaview Books, 1981.

BORG, SUSAN and LASKER, JUDITH. *When Pregnancy Fails: Families Coping with Miscarriage, Stillbirth and Infant Death*. Boston: Beacon Press, 1981.

FRIEDMAN, ROCHELLE and GRADSTEIN, BONNIE. *Surviving Pregnancy Loss*. Boston: Little, Brown and Co., 1981.

PIZER, HANK and PALINSKI, CHRISTINE O'BRIEN. *Coping with a Miscarriage*. New York: New American Library, 1980.

BOOKS ON ADOPTION

ANDERSON, DAVID C. *Children of Special Value*. New York: St. Martins Press, 1971.

BERMAN, CLAIRE. *We Take This Child*. New York: Doubleday & Co., 1974.

CANAPE, CHARLENE. *Adoption: Parenthood Without Pregnancy*. New York: Henry Holt and Co., 1986.

DULING, GRETCHEN. *Adopting Joe: A Black Vietnamese Child*. Rutland, Vermont: Charles E. Tuttle Co., 1977.

GILMAN, LOIS. *The Adoption Resources Book*. New York: Harper & Row, 1984.

KADUSHIN, ALFRED. *Adopting Older Children*. New York: Columbia University Press, 1970.

KLIBANOFF, SUSAN and KLIBANOFF, ELTON. *Let's Talk About Adoption*. Boston: Little, Brown and Co., 1973.

KRAMER, BETTY, ed. *The Unbroken Circle*. (A collection of writings on international and interracial adoption available from OURS, 3148 Humbolt Ave., S., Minneapolis, MN 55408.)

LADNER, JOYCE. *Mixed Families*. Garden City, New York: Anchor Press, 1977.

LIFTON, BETY JEAN. *Lost and Found: The Adoption Experience*. New York: The Dial Press, 1979.

MARGOLIES, MARJORIE and GRUBER, RUTH. *They Came Here to Stay*. New York: Coward, McCann and Geoghegan, Inc., 1976.

MACNAMERA, JOAN. *The Adoption Advisor*, Hawthorne Books, Inc., 1975.

MELINA, LOIS RUSKAI. *Raising Adopted Children: A Manual for Adoptive Parents*. New York: Harper & Row, 1986.

PLUMEZ, JACQUELINE H. *Successful Adoption: A Guide to Finding a Child and Raising a Family.* New York: Crown Publishers, 1982.

POWLEDGE, FRED. *The New Adoption Maze and How to Get Through It.* St. Louis: The C.V. Mosby Co., 1985.

SOROSKY, A., BARAN, A., and PANNOR, R. *The Adoption Triangle.* Garden City, New York: Anchor Press/Doubleday, 1978.

TAYLOR, MARY. *Intercountry Adoption Handbook.* (Available for $4 from Open Door Society of Massachusetts, 600 Washington Street, Boston, MA 02111.

VIGUERS, SUSAN. *With Child: One Couple's Journey to Their Adopted Children.* San Diego: Harcourt Brace Jovanovich, 1986.

BOOKS THAT DEAL WITH CHILD-FREE LIVING

DOWRICK, STEPHANIE and GRUNDBERG, SIBYL, eds. *Why Children?* New York: Harcourt Brace Jovanovich, 1980.

ELVENSTAR, DIANE C. *Children: To Have or Have Not?* San Francisco: Harbor Publishing, 1982.

PECK, ELLEN. *The Baby Trap.* New York: B. Geis Assoc., 1971.

PECK, ELLEN and SENDEROWITZ, JUDITH. *Pronatalism: The Myth of Mom and Apple Pie.* New York: Thomas Y. Crowell and Co., 1974.

WHELAN, ELIZABETH M. *A Baby? . . . Maybe.* New York: Bobbs-Merrill Co., 1975.

RESOURCES
AND
ORGANIZATIONS

MEDICAL ORGANIZATIONS

American College of Obstetrics and Gynecology
600 Maryland Avenue S.W., Suite 300
Washington, D.C. 20024

Professional medical organization for Ob-Gyns. Can provide names of
board-certified infertility specialists.

American Fertility Society
2131 Magnolia Avenue, Suite 201
Birmingham, AL 35256
(205) 933-7222

Professional organization for physicians interested in fertility and infertility.
Publishes monthly medical journal, *Fertility and Sterility*. Has booklets and
fact sheets available for sale at a nominal fee to the general public on
various aspects of infertility.

SELF-HELP ORGANIZATIONS

Compassionate Friends
P.O. Box 3696
Oak Brook, Ill. 60522
(312) 990-0010

A national self-help organization for bereaved parents and couples who have experienced pregnancy loss. Has 516 local chapters throughout the United States and publishes a newsletter.

Endometriosis Foundation
P.O. Box 92187
Milwaukee, WI 53202

Self-help organization with over 40 chapters. Publishes a newsletter.

RESOLVE, Inc.
5 Water Street
Arlington, MA 02174
(617) 643-2424

National self-help organization for infertile couples. Provides information, educational materials, referrals to fertility specialists; publishes a newsletter. Has over 40 local chapter and usually have support groups, counseling, and information and referral services.

National Organization for Nonparents
806 Reistertown Road
Baltimore, MD 21208

Organization that promotes and supports couples who choose to be child-free.

OTHER ORGANIZATIONS WITH NEWSLETTERS

Center for Communications in Infertility, Inc.
P.O. Box 516
Yorktown Heights, NY 10508

Publishes a bimonthly newsletter, *Perspectives on Infertility*, and provides information on infertility.

SURROGATE PARENTING NEWS
120 North Fourth Avenue
Ann Arbor, MI 48104

A monthly newsletter about surrogate motherhood and related subjects.

ADOPTION RESOURCES

Child Welfare League of America
440 First Avenue NW
Washington, DC 20001
(202) 638-2952

National policy and standard-setting agency in the field of child welfare services. Provides information about agency and independent (private) adoption for prospective parents and professionals.

International Alliance for Children, Inc.
2 Ledge Lane
New Milford, Connecticut
(203) 354-3417

Latin American Parents Association (LAPA)
P.O. Box 72
Seaford, NY 11783
(516) 783-6942

A national organization with branches in six states.

National Adoption Exchange
1218 Chestnut Street, Suite 404
Philadelphia, PA 19107
(215) 925-0200

Agency with adoption listings all over the country. Mostly "special needs" children.

North American Council on Adoptable Children (NACAC)
250 East Blaine
Riverside, CA 92507

North American Council on Adoptable Children
2001 South Street NW, Suite 540
Washington, DC 20009
(202) 466-7570

North American Council on Adoptable Children
P.O. Box 14808
Minneapolis, MN 55414

Has newsletter, *ADOPTALK*, and other publications on adoption.

Open Door Society of Massachusetts, Inc.
600 Washington Street
Boston, Massachusetts 02111

Has newsletter and other publications on adoption.

OURS, Inc.
4711 30th Avenue South
Minneapolis, MN 55406

Has newsletter and other publications on adoption.

Parents for Private Adoption
P.O. Box 7
Pawlet, VT 05761

Provides information and newsletter on legal, private adoption.

BREAST-FEEDING ADOPTED CHILDREN

Lact-Aid International, Inc.
P.O. Box 10066
Athens, TN 37303
(615) 744-9090

La Leche League International
P.O. Box 1209
Franklin Park, Illinois 60131-8209

La Leche League has local branches in many cities.

IN VITRO FERTILIZATION CLINICS

There are over 200 *in vitro* fertilization clinics in United States alone. The American Fertility Society or RESOLVE can give you the names in your area that meet minimal standards.

SURROGATE MOTHER SERVICES

(This list is for information only and does not imply the author's endorsement.)

CALIFORNIA

Center for Surrogate Parenting
8383 Wilshire Blvd., Suite 750

Beverly Hills, CA 90211
(213) 655-1974

The Surrogate Parent Program
11110 Ohio Avenue, Suite 202
Los Angeles, CA 90025
(213) 473-8961

Surrogate Parent Foundation, Inc.
12345 Oxnard Street
North Hollywood, CA 91606
(213) 506-1804

The Hagar Institute
401 Marina Blvd., Suite 125
South San Francisco, CA 94080
(415) 873-8818

KANSAS

The Hagar Institute
1015 Buchanan
Topeka, KS 66604

KENTUCKY

Surrogate Family Services, Inc.
125 South Seventh Street
Louisville, KY 40202

Surrogate Parenting Associates, Inc.
250 E. Liberty Street
Louisville, KY 40202
(502) 584-7794

MARYLAND

National Center for Surrogate Parenting
5530 Wisconsin Avenue
Chevy Chase, MD 20815

MICHIGAN

Noel Keane, J.D.
930 Mason
Dearborn, MI 48124

Genesearch
757 Oakdale Avenue
Jackson, MI 49208
(517) 789-7310

Ames Center for Surrogate Parenting, Inc.
P.O. Box 9201
Livonia, MI 48150

NEW YORK

Buffalo Infertility Center
5285 Chestnut Ridge Road
Orchard Park, NY 14127
(716) 662-9041

The Infertility Center of New York
14 East 60th Street, Suite 1204
New York, NY 10022
(212) 371-0811

OHIO

Association for Surrogate Parenting Services, Inc.
42 South
Philadelphia, PA 19102

ORGANIZATIONS FOR LEGAL ACTION

DES Action—East Coast Branch
Long Island Jewish Hillside Medical Center
New Hyde Park, NY 10040
(516) 775-3450

DES Action—West Coast Branch
2845 24th Street
San Francisco, CA 94110

National nonprofit organization that provides medical and legal information for DES victims.

IUD Litigation Resource
Litigation Information Service
National Women's Health Network
224 Seventh Street S.E.
Washington, DC 20003

Legal advice for women whose infertility is due to an IUD, especially the Dalkon shield.

INDEX

Abortions, 4, 14

Adoption, 63, 70, 131, 147–64
  agency, dealing with, 154–57, 158
  books on, 177–78
  breast-feeding adopted child, 149, 184
  consideration of, 123–25, 126–27, 154
  counseling regarding, 151
  decision to adopt, 152–53, 154
  emotions regarding, 149–53, 160–61
  fantasizing about, 130
  fears regarding 147–50
  marital conflicts regarding, 150–51, 160–61
  organizations and resources, 183–84
  physical appearance of baby, 161–62, 163
  positive feelings, 152–53, 162–64
  pregnancy following, 109, 110–11, 152
  private adoption, 148–49, 184
  race of baby, 147, 154, 158–59
  receiving the child, 158–64
  time factors, 148, 158

Age of couples, 4, 9

American Fertility Society, 21, 22, 32, 34, 113, 132–33

Andrews, Lori B., 136

Andrologists, 20

Anger, 43–45, 46
  pregnant women, reactions to, 73–80
  of wives, 42, 45

Anxiety, 27, 28–29
  donor insemination (AID), regarding, 136–45
  first failures at conception, 2–3, 5–6, 8, 13–15
  husbands, 6, 8
  switching doctors, 34–36
  wives, 2–3, 5–6

Artificial insemination
  with donor sperm (AID), 97–98, 99, 128, 131, 133–36, 136–45
  husband's (AIH), 18, 27, 37, 39, 89, 92, 108–109

Baby M Case, 131

Bacterial infections, 12, 38

ABOUT THE AUTHOR

JOAN LIEBMANN-SMITH is a medical sociologist and a freelance writer. She has a Masters Degree in sociology from the Graduate Center of the City University of New York, where she is presently working on her doctoral thesis on delayed childbearing and infertility. She has been involved with infertility both academically and personally; during 1981–1982 she was co-president of the New York City chapter of RESOLVE, a national self-help organization for infertile couples.

Ms. Liebmann-Smith has written on health topics for national magazines, including *Vogue, Self, American Health*, and *MS. In Pursuit of Pregnancy* is her first book. She lives in New York City with her husband, Richard, who is a writer and editor, and their four-year-old daughter, Rebecca.